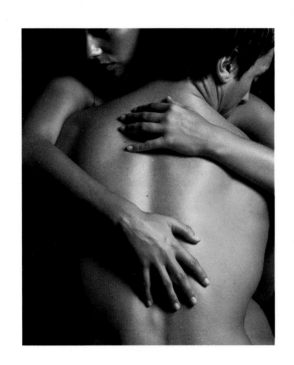

super**hot**sex

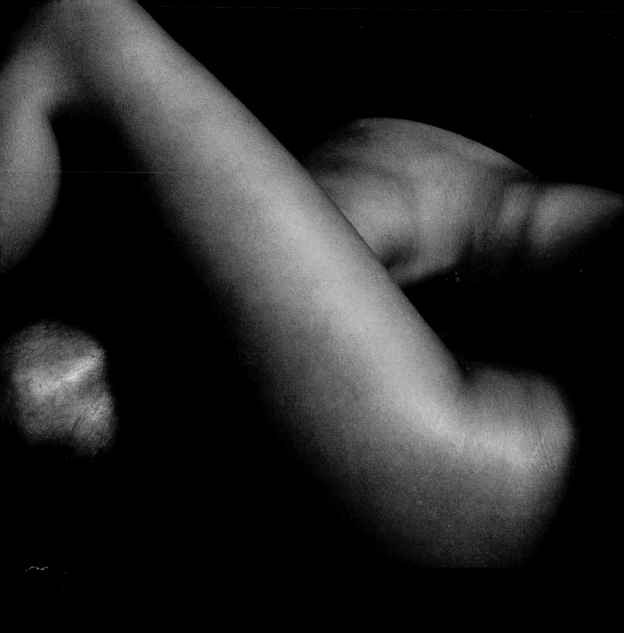

photography by John Davis

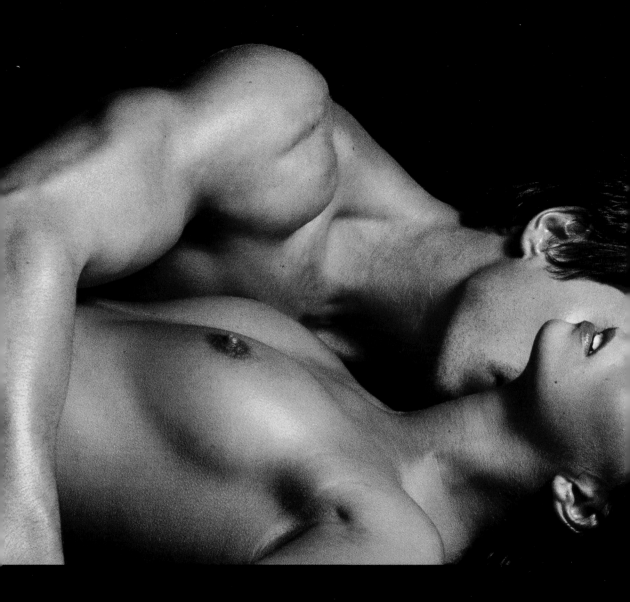

superhotsex

tracey cox

LONDON, NEW YORK, MUNICH,
MELBOURNE, DELHI

Editor Dawn Bates
Design XAB Design
Senior Editor Salima Hirani
Senior Art Editor Nicola Rodway
Executive Managing Editor Adèle Hayward
Managing Art Editor Karla Jennings
DTP Designer Traci Salter
Production Controller Luca Frassinetti
Art Director Peter Luff
Publishing Director Corinne Roberts

First American Edition, 2006
Published in the United States by DK Publishing, Inc.,
375 Hudson Street, New York, NY 10014

06 07 08 09 10   10 9 8 7 6 5 4 3 2 1

ISBN-10: 0-7566-2275-1
ISBN-13: 978-0-7566-2275-6

DK books are available at special discounts for bulk
purchases for sales promotions, premiums, fund-
raising, or educational use. For details, contact:
DK Publishing Special Markets, 375 Hudson Street,
New York, NY 10014 or SpecialSales@dk.com

Reproduced by Colourscan, Singapore
Printed and bound by Tien Wah Press, Singapore

Always practice safe and responsible sex,
and consult a doctor if you have any condition
that might preclude strenuous sexual activity.
The author and publisher do not accept any
responsibility for any injury or ailment caused
by following any of the suggestions contained in
this book. They would also like to remind readers
that the law takes a dim view of people exposing
themselves in public or offending others; always
be discreet (and avoid getting arrested!).

Discover more at **www.dk.com**

Contents

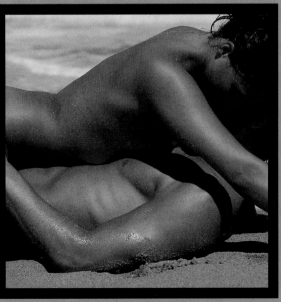

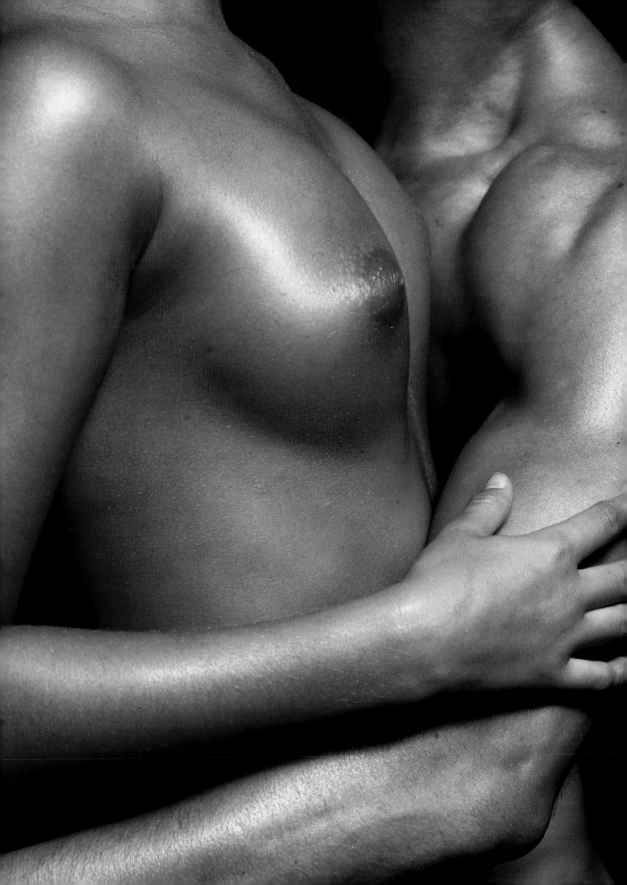

Introduction

For most of us, sex isn't a problem at the start of a relationship. Everything is new, you're both aiming to please, and pleasure is delivered daily by the truckload. New flesh is a seductive aphrodisiac and sexual satisfaction something you take for granted. Falling asleep, hands clamped to each other's naughty parts and smug smiles on your faces, you're convinced you'll be different from the rest. Of course you can have great sex five, ten, even twenty years from now! .... Except just two years later, those same hands have found new targets to wrap around—coffee cups—and instead of devouring each other, it's the latest bestseller. You're content, happy even, but can't help but feel ever so slightly cheated. Like, *what the hell happened to our sex life?*

Is there anything that can beat *really really good sex?* True, chocolate, shopping, football, and pizza come **a close second** for some, but **sex** will never be knocked off **the Number One spot**.

This book is for anyone who's ever wondered why sex is sooooo easy in the beginning but increasingly difficult the more time you spend together. Those of you who've read *supersex* know the basics and have no doubt mastered more than a few techniques. You're sexually confident— which makes it even more frustrating when things aren't as good as you sense they could be. *superhotsex* aims not only to help you get back the fantastic sex you used to have, it's designed to take your sex life to another level. By getting you to be much more sexually adventurous, I intend to push you (very gently) out of (boring) sexual comfort zones and into (exciting, exhilarating) new modes of thinking and behaving. Yes, you might have to make a bit of an effort, but by God, it's going to be worth it! Cast your mind back. Is there anything on this planet that can beat *really really r-e-a-l-l-y good sex?* True, chocolate, shopping, football, and pizza come a close second for some, but sex will never be knocked off the Number One spot. It's powerful stuff. Powerful enough to make kings give up their thrones, the rich hand over their fortunes, and sensible career women go so limp with lust, they'll give up fabulous jobs they've worked years for, to follow some temperamental lover who wants to "find himself" in Kathmandu.

Want more or better sex? (And doesn't everyone?) Turn the page and start reading.
You might just find you're having superhotsex—for life!

Tracey X

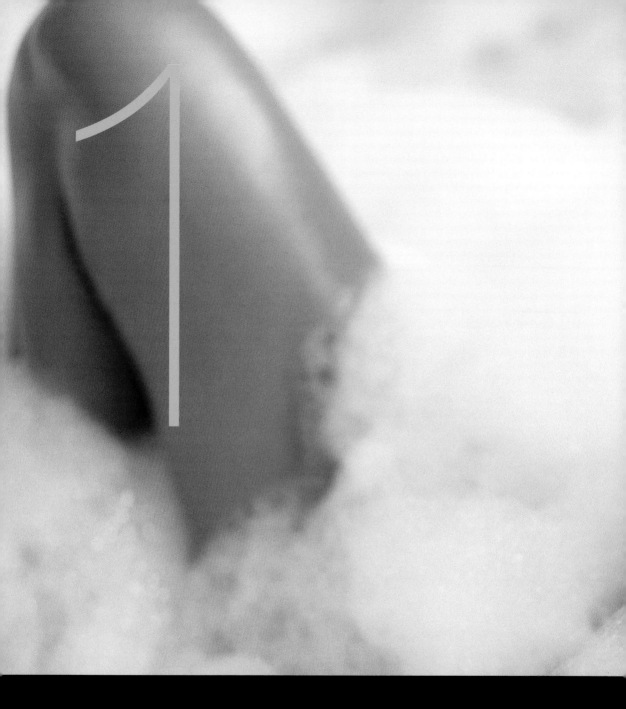

1

The secret ingredients for sensational long-term sex, and why there are NO excuses for not cooking up a continual carnal feast!

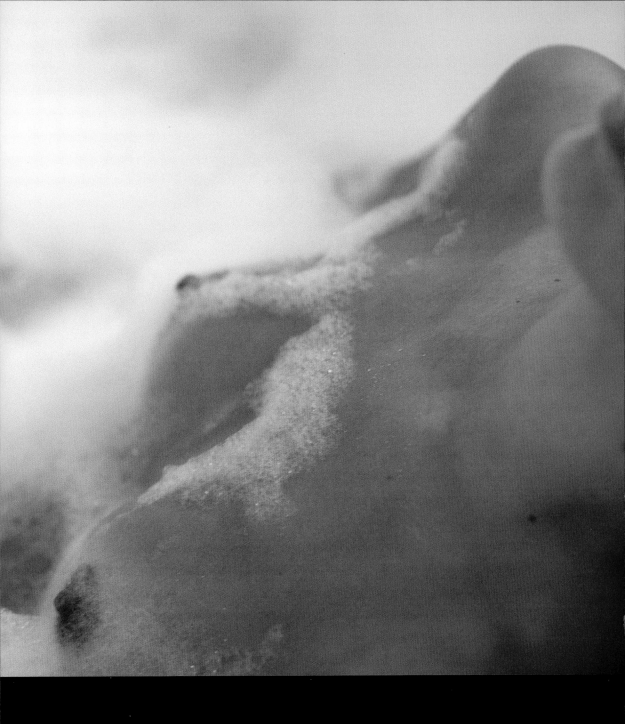

Come on, you know
you want to!

Two in a tub

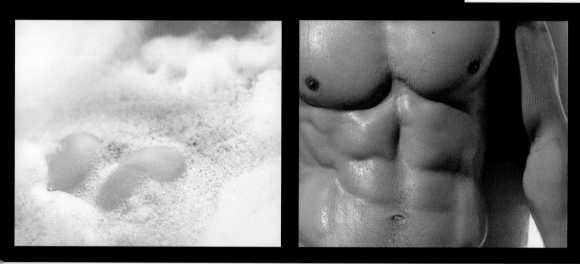

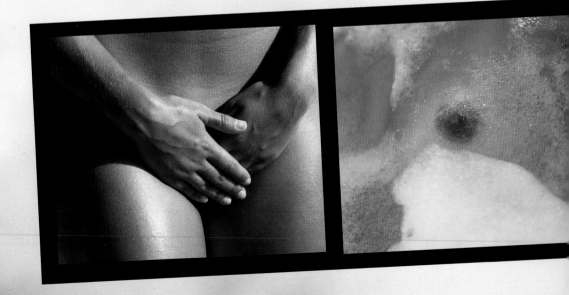

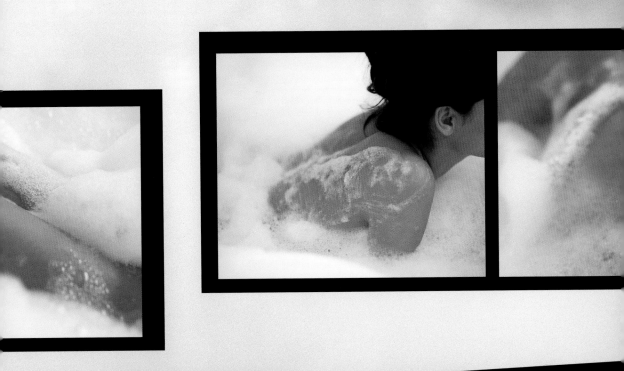

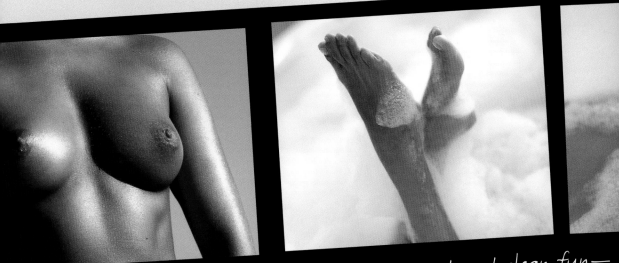

Bubbles are playful, provocative, and good clean fun—which becomes anything but when two share a tub.

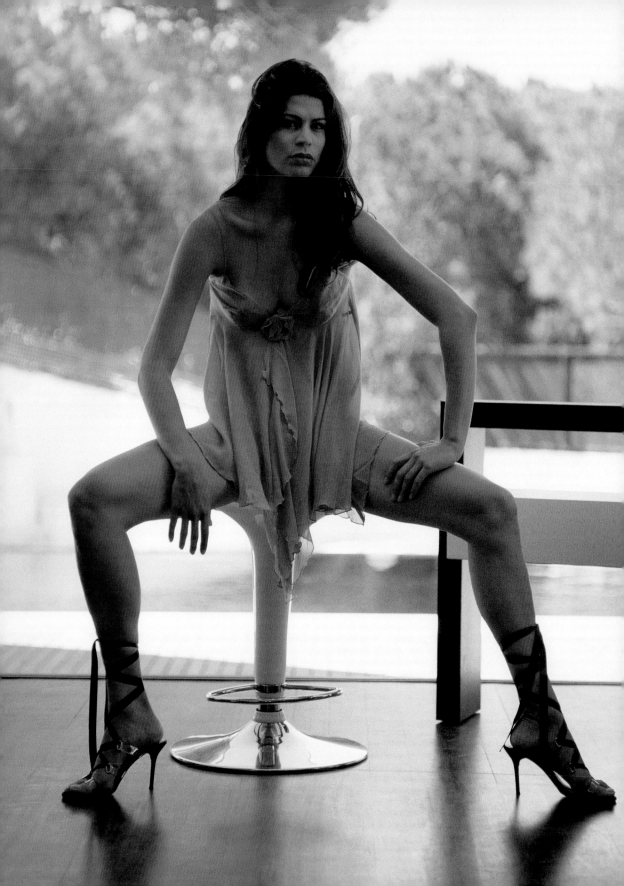

Lust to last a lifetime
How to future-proof your sex life

Sex isn't important. It might be in the beginning, but long-term love isn't about lust, it's about love, friendship, and commitment. If we were all brutally honest and stopped kidding ourselves, we'd accept that as long as you're having some type of sex with your partner, you're actually doing OK. Sure, you might feel the occasional twinge of jealousy when you watch couples who've just hooked up, but kids, friends, being part of a family, having someone to support you, to rely on, and to snuggle up to at night more than makes up for the lack of lust.

Does the girl opposite look like she'd put up with a lifetime of mediocre sex?
Then why should you? Don't settle—aim high!

No, you haven't picked up the wrong book; this is what a good majority of long-term couples believe. And there's nothing wrong with thinking like this—if you're prepared to accept mediocre sex as your lot in life. If you don't even blink at that statement, by all means continue to think like that (and hope like hell your partner agrees with you). If, on the other hand, the thought of a lifetime of so-so sex makes you want to stick your head in the nearest gas oven, you may find this book interesting (not to mention the rest of your relationship).

GREED IS GOOD

I don't think there are any prizes for guessing which camp I fall into. I'm a greedy bugger—I want it all. I want the kind of intimacy, contentment, deep affection, and security only long-term love brings. But I also want passion, lust, eroticism, and spontaneity. I am well aware the two often aren't bedfellows, but I'm also not completely deluded! These days, we're so brow-beaten by "experts" telling us we expect too much from sex and relationships, anyone who's still trumpeting high ideals gets a nasty rap across the knuckles. (Naughty! How dare you expect to be happy in bed and out!) But relationships like the one I'm describing do exist—and not just in my head after a dozen drinks. True, you probably won't haphazardly stumble across one taking the dog for its

One out of every three couples struggles with problems associated with low sexual desire. One study found 20 percent of married couples have sex fewer than ten times a year.

Want to end up like these guys—so bored you can't wait for sex to be over? **Good sex that lasts isn't a gift, it's an achievement.**

five-minute walk tonight, but I bet if you tried you could think of a few lucky so-and-so's you've met. So if you want a great sex life as well as (shock! horror!) a good relationship, let's applaud your optimism rather than deflate it, by looking at how you can add your names to this exclusive list.

It pays to aim high! Couples who have regular, good sex aren't just the happiest, they tend to have the highest libidos. Sex stimulates the production of testosterone, so the more sex you have, the more you want. It keeps us healthy and energetic, which helps get us in the mood; it boosts immunity, warding off colds and infections; and sexually active people also appear to be less susceptible to depression and suicide. Orgasms could even be life-extending, most likely because of the effects on the heart and immune system. So sex is good for your body, your mental health, *and* your relationship!

SO WHAT'S THE SECRET?

What, then, do you have to do to become one of those enviable long-term couples who eagerly anticipate sex, rather than try their damnedest to avoid it? While it's all individual, there are definitely common themes. Anyone who's read any of my other books knows I consider understanding the

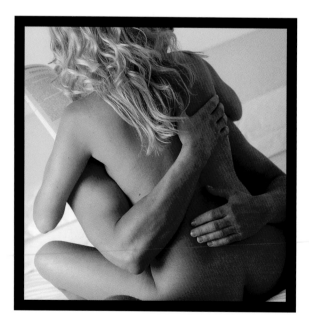

mechanics of sex and mastering effective techniques crucial cornerstones to a great sex life. These are definitely essential. But there's something else that appears to be even more important—in fact, without it, the other things are immaterial: arousal. Arousal appears to be the key ingredient needed to drive good, long-term sex. It's the pursuit of pleasure, after all, that makes us want to have sex in the first place. If you're not aroused, your motivation to have sex is low or nonexistent. Plunking your butt on the couch, remote in hand, is a more attractive option because even the tamest, lamest sexual experience requires some emotional and physical energy. If you're not aroused emotionally or physically, where does that

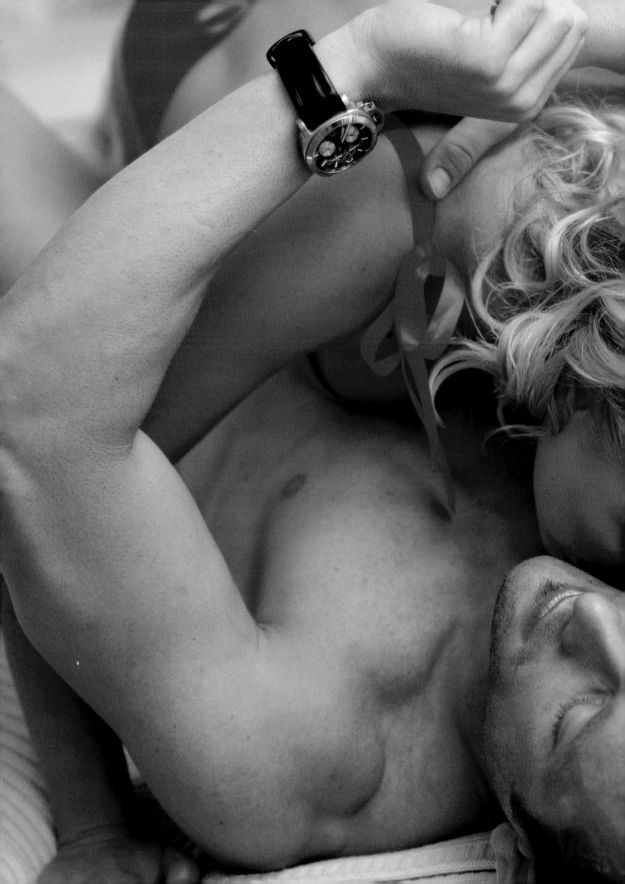

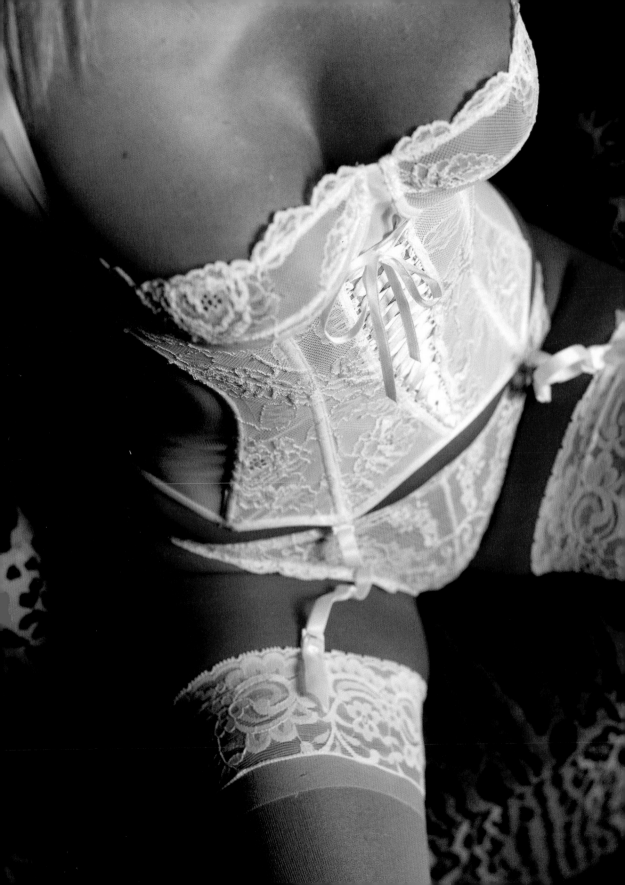

Studies show people who have **sex 4–5 times a week** look **10 years younger** than those who clock up the twice-a-week average.

energy come from? And how do some couples manage to remain aroused while the rest don't? It requires a level of openness and honesty that most people aren't used to. Along with high arousal levels, sexually satisfied couples are sexually adventurous—the two, in fact, feed each other. Satisfied couples pay attention to the cliché that says you need to do new things to spice up your sex life, but they don't opt for the standard suggestions of what that might be (e.g., candles, massage, and a pair of new panties). Their idea of "new things" includes raunchy, risky activities the average couple would gulp at and consider "inappropriate."

"GROWN-UP" SEX ISN'T SUPPOSED TO BE NAUGHTY

A hell of a lot of couples think married or long-term sex is supposed to be loving and affectionate, and feel guilty for craving the "nasty" or "dirty" sex they enjoyed while single (or in their imaginations). If you truly love your partner, the need to keep them in love with you can stop you from doing or suggesting anything that might damage that. Being able to get past that vulnerability and not be scared to show what you really want sexually is a key factor for success. If you're not crippled by the need for your partner to approve of every sexual need and feeling you have, you're far more likely to be daring. We want our partners to reassure us that everything we do and say is "normal," but by doing so, we stop ourselves from letting those slightly odd (more interesting) urges and cravings surface. Couples who enjoy lusty sex long-term have broken through these barriers. They might not like everything their partner says or does, or enjoy every sexual experience they try, but they feel a sense of sexual freedom that is conspicuously absent from your "average" (read "so-so" sex) relationship.

Good technique. Arousal. Being sexually adventurous. Openness and honesty. These are our themes. Now explore them with me (I promise we'll take baby steps!) and set yourself up for lust that will last a lifetime.

Not in the mood?
"Forcing yourself" to have sex when you don't feel like it sounds dreadful, but I've seen miraculous effects on people's sex drive because of it. What initially seems like an effort can have a pleasant effect—and there's evidence that putting effort into rejuvenating one area will breathe new life into your whole relationship. Give it a try. (Come on, it's not like I'm asking you to devour a plate of raw liver!)

Excuses, excuses, excuses
There are none!

You're anticipating a feisty frolic, one hand hovering over your zipper, and they say... "No." OK, not quite what the sex therapist ordered, but never fear, help is at hand! It's natural to be a little resistant to change, so here are a few hints on how to talk around a reluctant partner or give yourself courage.

I'm too old for that

If you can still eat, breathe, and smile, you can still be open to new sexual experiences. Age is mainly an attitude. I appreciate that health problems and aging can influence which ideas or techniques you choose, but disregarding new things just because you think they're for "young" people is silly. Assuming you're not parking a walker next to your lover's scooter, you're probably around the same age. So if it's your body you're worried about, I'll bet theirs isn't perfect either. Adventurous sex isn't something only the young indulge in, so start living rather than waiting to die. (A bit harsh, I know, but come on!)

I'm happy with how things are/so-so sex

Many people really don't want great sex. Passionate sex is physically and emotionally powerful, and if you don't like losing control, it's appalling rather than appealing. Intense sex usually means an intense relationship, and that means intense pain if it all goes horribly wrong. If you've been burned in the past and don't subscribe to the "better to have loved and lost" theory, you might want to play it safe. Other people simply have a naturally low libido and can't really understand what all the fuss is about. If both of you are truly content to laze around in So-So Sex Land, not wanting to change isn't a problem, and you shouldn't feel any pressure to. There is a problem, however, if only one of you feels this way, because mismatched sexual expectation and/or fulfillment leaves you wide open to an affair.

What about the kids?

Assuming you're not planning to put on a floor show at bedtime/use the baby's pacifier for unhygienic purposes/lock the kids in the attic for a few days to avoid being interrupted, there are ways around the child problem. Get a babysitter when you feel like trying something special, and time quick sex sessions for when they're engrossed in their favorite TV show. Make friends with other parents so you can take turns watching the kids, and put a radio beside your bed to drown out the moans. If (ohmigod, they'll be scarred forever!) the kids do catch you in the act, don't panic. If they're little, explain calmly that Mommy and Daddy were doing what adults do when they're grown up and in love/married. If they're older, they'll probably be more embarrassed than you are

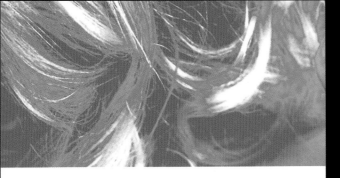

and will have rushed out of the room and slammed the door before their brain has even formed the word "Gross!". Avoid the awkward post-discovery moment by using it as a springboard to have that birds-and-bees talk or put some good, nonjudgmental and informative sex books in their room—"just in case" they need them.

I'm just not the adventurous type

We all have different personalities, and while some people hate routine, others love it. Extroverts tend to welcome change, introverts dislike it—usually because their confidence level is lower. The more secure you are, the more likely you are to try new things because the risks are low. If you fail or make a fool of yourself, so what? Your self-esteem and ego can take the occasional dent. If you're the one wanting adventure, reassure your partner that it's OK to take baby steps and you'll hold their hand all the way. Also make it clear that you'll stop if they don't like it.

I'm too shy/I'd feel embarrassed

Worrying that you'll feel like a complete twit during role-play, look decidedly unsexy in that nurse's outfit, or just get it "wrong" are natural fears. If you're not a person who's comfortable in the spotlight, being tied up naked with legs and arms splayed probably isn't going to make you feel like your ship has just come in. The trick to getting through it is to start with the thing you find least scary and work up to doing the others. If you're not an exhibitionist, there may be things you'll never enjoy. In those cases, let your partner take the dominant role.

The secrets of successful sex

- **Variety:** Try three new intercourse positions every three months; try at least one new sex "act" per month; vary the order, length of time, and techniques of foreplay each and every session. (Accomplish this by turning off the television.)

- **Quantity:** Aim to have a minimum of three quick sex sessions and two longer sessions per month. (Again, turn off the boob tube and time will magically appear.)

- **Communication:** Teach yourselves to talk openly and honestly about your needs and wants. Make a pact never to judge anything your partner suggests.

- **Education:** Buy at least two sex books a year and look for articles that keep you abreast of new research.

- **Erotica:** Watch sexy movies, read sexy books, look at sexy images. Focusing on sex keeps your libido high. (You can turn the TV on for this one!)

- **Affection:** Kissing your partner for just 20 seconds every day could mean the difference between make or break for your relationship. Touch, kiss, and cuddle out of bed, not just in it. (TV allowed as long as you snuggle on the same couch.)

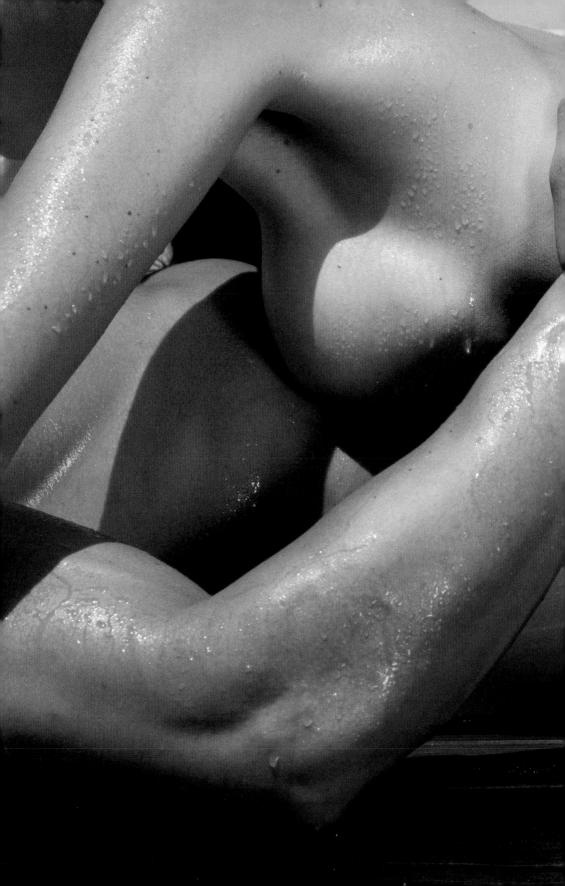

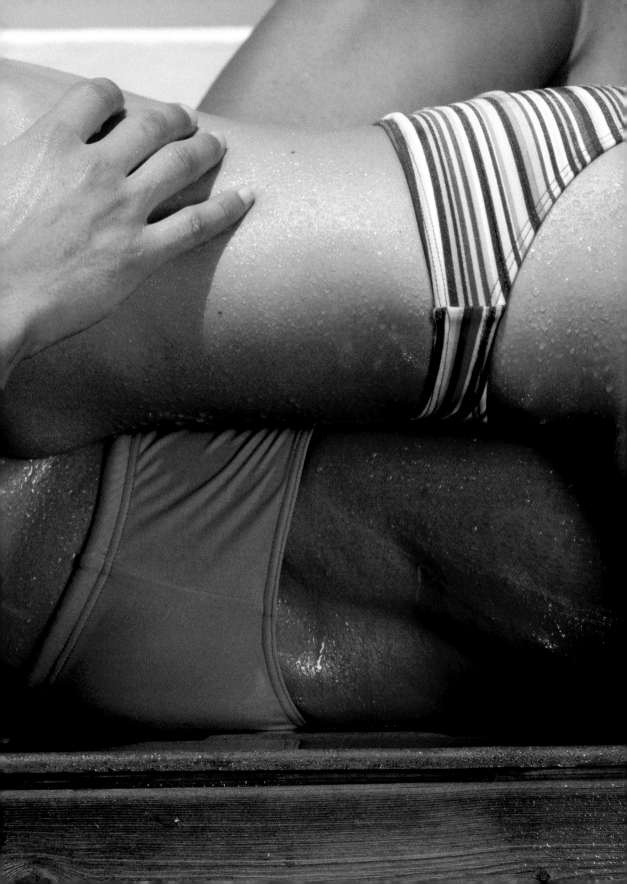

Orgasm masterclass
A lust lesson for him

I've written this feature especially for men, so you can understand her body better and help even up the orgasm ratio (which currently stands at around three [yours] to one [hers], if she's lucky and you're a great lover). You won't find the equivalent story for her because there's no need. Here's why:

A recent British study found that **80 percent of women fake orgasms during intercourse.** In the US, **53 percent** of women said they **prefer shopping to sex**.

Your penis and sexual system is gloriously, wonderfully simple. The penis—the organ that needs stimulation to produce a male orgasm—is designed to go inside the vagina, where it's all warm and snug. Thrusting during intercourse provides the friction needed to stimulate the nerve endings and before you can say, "Oh God, I think I'm... ", you normally have. Women's bodies are complicated. Quite frankly, whoever designed us appears to have been far too focused on the baby part, with far too little attention given to the making of it.

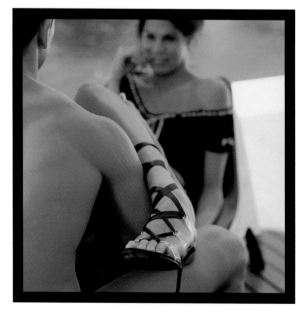

The clitoris—the organ we need stimulated to produce an orgasm—isn't inside the vagina where it should be, but stuck a distance away. Since intercourse is usually the "main event" for most couples, it's left looking on in bewilderment, wondering why it hasn't been invited to the party. Sadly, this design fault can't be corrected the same way your iPod would, if the wheel in the middle proved to be a pain in the ass position-wise. We're stuck with it—and so are you. This doesn't mean women are destined for a dreadful time in bed, while you lucky devils live it up. It just means you need to pay more attention to her orgasm than your own.

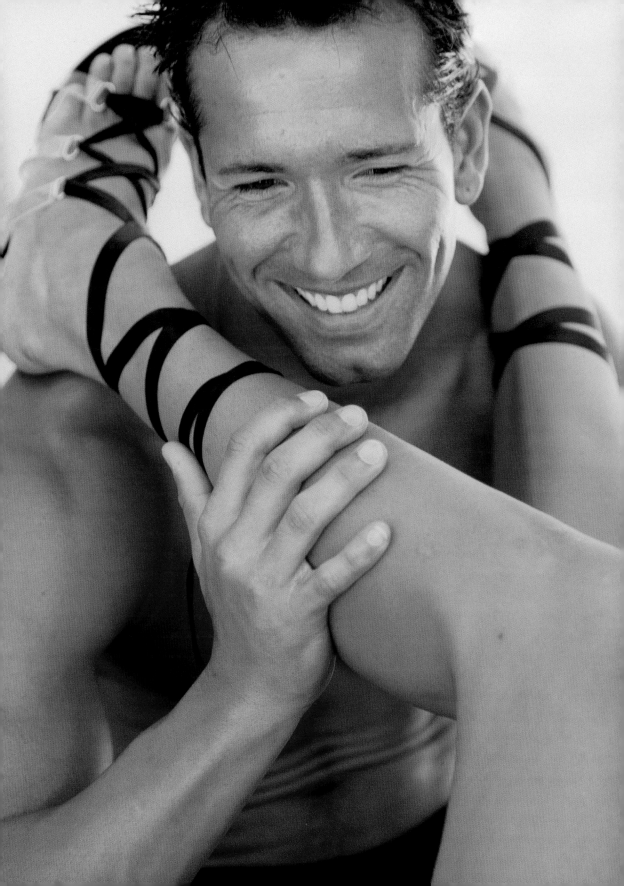

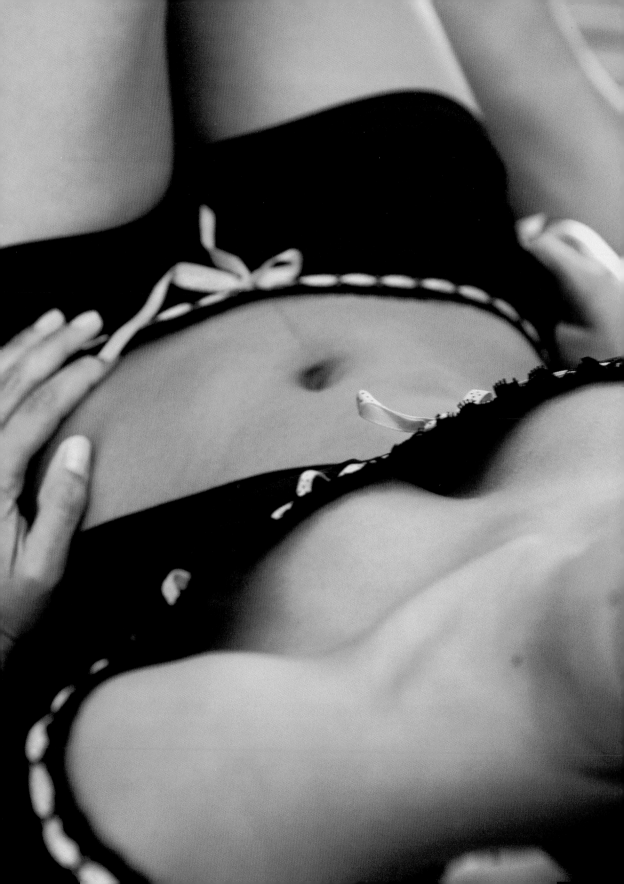

There's lots of research into female orgasm. Debate continues over whether there is only one female orgasm (clitoral) or others (vaginal, "blended"—achieved through simultaneous vaginal and clitoral stimulation—or G-spot). Nearly all the "serious" sex experts (sex therapists, sexologists, etc.) state clearly that all female orgasms are triggered by stimulation of the clitoris. Other "sexperts"—and women who aren't—claim there are other ways a woman climaxes that don't involve the clitoris at all. From my experience writing and researching sex, I tend to agree with the white-coat brigade.

Since intercourse is usually "the main event," **the clitoris is left looking on, wondering why it hasn't been asked to the party!**

For most women, the clitoris must come into direct contact with something for us to orgasm. But this doesn't mean it's impossible to orgasm during penetration alone. For about one-third of all women, your thrusting inside the vagina can create enough stimulation on the clitoris and the adjacent area to produce an orgasm from intercourse alone. One theory is that these women have a larger-than-usual clitoris, or one positioned closer to the vaginal opening than normal. Another is that it's achieved with men who use a grinding motion. Others manage to climax from penetration alone by getting themselves stimulated to the brink of orgasm and use thrusting as a final trigger to push them over the edge. So if she's to climax, you need to think beforehand about what's likely to do it for her—don't just assume it will happen. Spanking, fantasy, role-play, phone sex, a cheek-reddening visit to a swinger's club (more on these later): all are fabulous for arousal and upping the intensity and eroticism of the experience so she's far closer to orgasm. But you may still have to give the clitoris a twirl around the dance floor before you can both do a congratulatory dip.

Don't forget about the basics, just because you're trying new stuff.

The clitoris isn't the only thing getting attention in the research labs. If you want to really impress her, take a tip from recent studies into pelvic muscle control and their effect on orgasm. Traditionally, women have been told to pull in and tighten their pelvic muscles just before orgasm, to ensure a better experience for both of you. Now there's evidence that doing the opposite—pushing them out—could make orgasm more intense. My advice on who to believe? Try everything and let her make up her own mind about what works for her!

Two-thirds of women surveyed by a popular website said sex with their partner improved over time, once he "got to know" her body.

ORGASM ESSENTIALS
• Good-quality lubricants

Under ideal circumstances, her body produces enough natural lubrication not to warrant adding any extra—"ideal" meaning she's healthy, not stressed, it's the right time of the month, she doesn't have a hangover, hasn't drunk too much or taken any antihistamines to dry up that runny nose (they dry everything else up, too), and is feeling happy, relaxed, and aroused. Which, let's face it, is about one day in twenty. Adding artificial moisture—in the form of a good-quality personal lubricant—is a sensible way of making sure sex feels pleasurable for both of you. But it's not just useful during penetration. If you're using your hands and fingers on yourself or her, lubrication means you can maintain a nice, even, steady rhythm because your hands glide more freely with added moisture. Keep a tube or bottle near the bed to squeeze on the appropriate parts when necessary.

Does orgasm feel the same for men and women? When researchers asked both sexes to write a detailed description, the judges couldn't tell the difference.

• A vibrator

Vibrators aren't just for women—really. As a man, you probably assume they're used purely by women to masturbate with, and happily leave her to it. Besides, they're scary-looking things! The old-fashioned style of vibrators *were* pretty scary: ten inches long with throbbing, lifelike veins, and made of squishy, horrible stuff that looked alarmingly like a penis. Except much bigger and much longer and much wider and... *ohmigod, is that what women really want?* The answer is no. The old-style penislike vibrators were designed by men—men who, sadly, didn't have much idea of what women wanted. Look at most successful vibrator ranges today (see page 111)—nearly all heavily influenced by women—and the first thing you'll notice is that most aren't even penis-shaped. They're designed to stimulate the clitoris, rather than for penetration. Yes, the "Rabbit"—made famous by *Sex and the City*—is a firm favorite, but plenty of women turn it around and simply use the clitoral stimulator rather than insert it. They've become more clitoris-focused because few women can orgasm purely through penetration with no clitoral stimulation. Which means one of you usually has to use your fingers to stimulate the clitoris during intercourse. This is harder than it sounds. It's awkward—your hand gets cramped—and it's hard to keep the gentle, consistent pressure the clitoris needs when your hand is being pushed by the thrusting motion. The solution is a small wand-style vibrator. One of you holds it against the clitoral area during intercourse and *voila!*, an orgasm during penetration. For your pleasure, get her to hold it against her mouth during oral sex and hold it against your hand while you're masturbating.

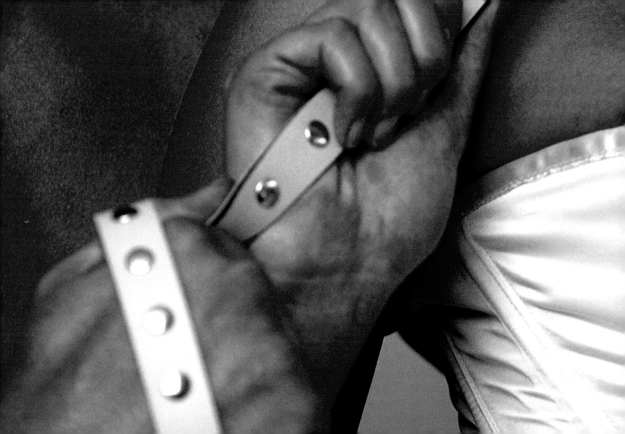

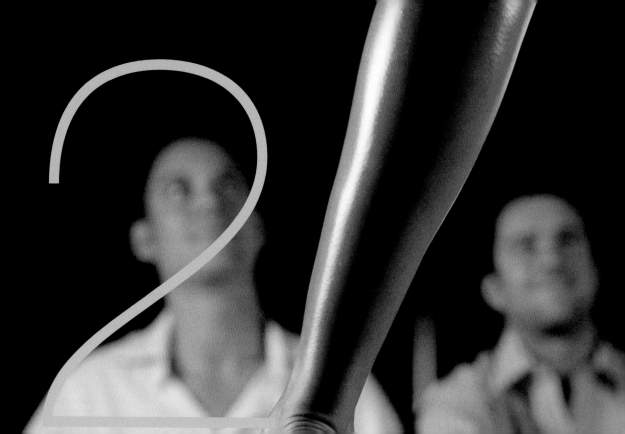

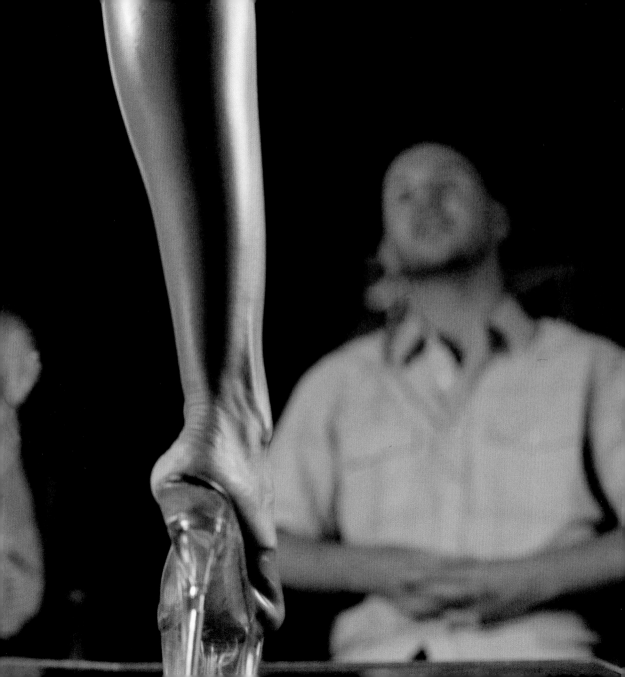

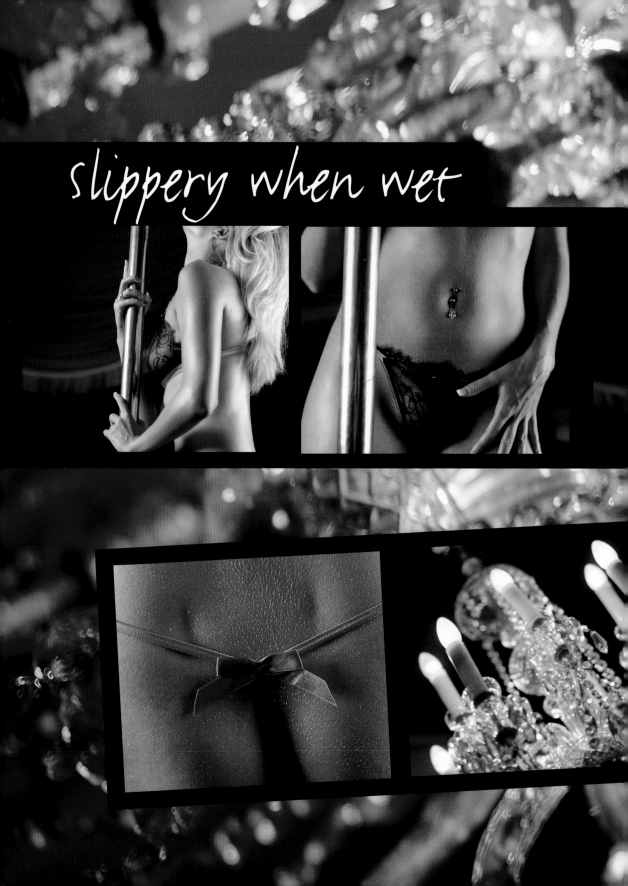

slippery when wet

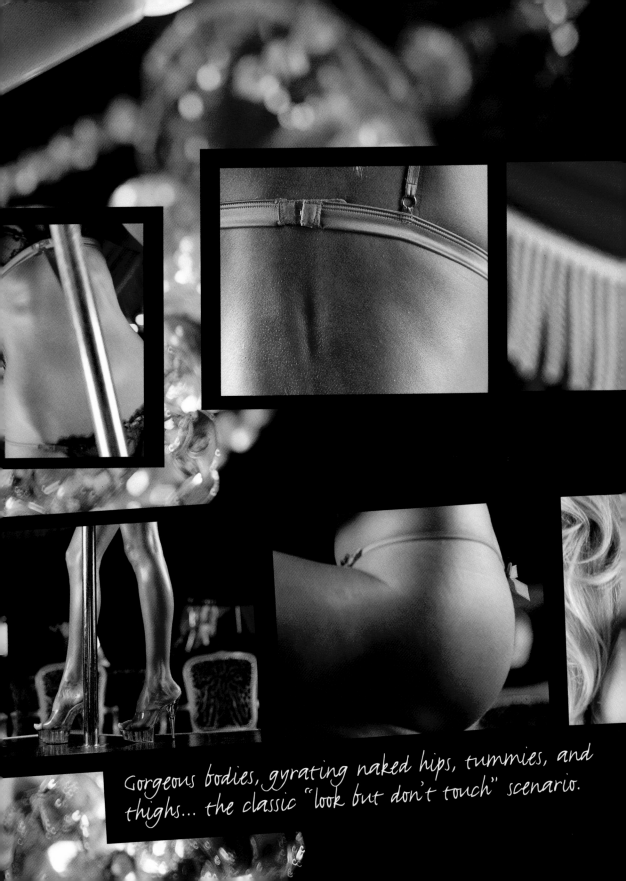

Gorgeous bodies, gyrating naked hips, tummies, and thighs... the classic "look but don't touch" scenario.

Head sex

Why wicked thoughts about others can save the relationship you're in

You want them. You can't stop thinking about them. If you don't have them, you're going to spontaneously combust with pent-up lust. Just one minor problem: the person you've got your eye on just happens to be your wife's best friend/your boyfriend's father/your boss. And it probably wouldn't be great if your partner found out. To put it mildly. It's an impossible situation that is making

> We're all **drawn to the "dark side" of sexuality.** We might wrinkle our noses and brand **lap dancers and strippers** distasteful when in polite company, but you can bet **your next orgasm** they've **featured heavily in fantasy land.**

you squirm for all sorts of reasons. Want my advice on what to do? Go ahead and indulge, and to hell with the consequences! Invite the best friend over under some flimsy pretext, ply her with gin and tonic, then confess the wicked X-rated daydream she stars in. Smile back at that hot-looking girl who got on the bus and (come on, that was deliberate!) flashed you a glimpse of her (black, lacy) panties. Get off at her stop. Follow her and have raw, animal sex up against a wall in a deserted parking ramp. Take a nice cold beer over to the gorgeous man painting your neighbor's fence. Say you couldn't help but notice his great muscles, with his shirt off and all. Then take him up on his offer to feel how hard they are, let your fingers linger a little, meet his eyes, and answer the unspoken invitation by asking him inside. In fact, go right ahead and have sex with whoever you want, whenever you want—all at once, if you wish! There's only one rule I want to enforce: all the action happens in your head. (And please, God, tell me you kept reading till you got to this part, rather than rushing out the door immediately.)

Feeling slightly conned? Don't be. You'd be surprised how effective fantasy is for satisfying a sexual itch. You get all the pleasure without the pain of broken hearts and failed relationships.

For him, sex worker fantasies are pure, lusty, selfish sex without morals or consequence. For her, they're proof she's attractive; if he's willing to pay for it, she must be good...

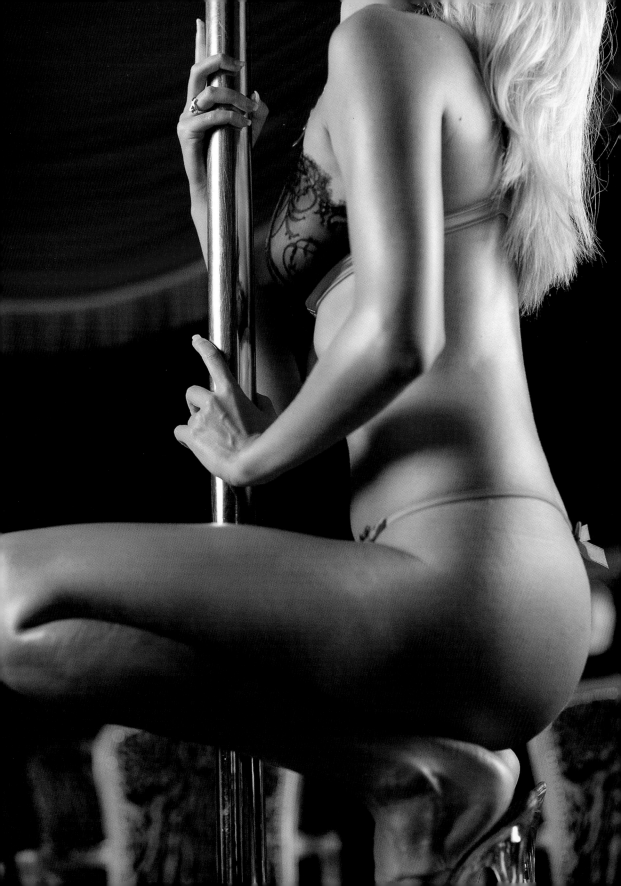

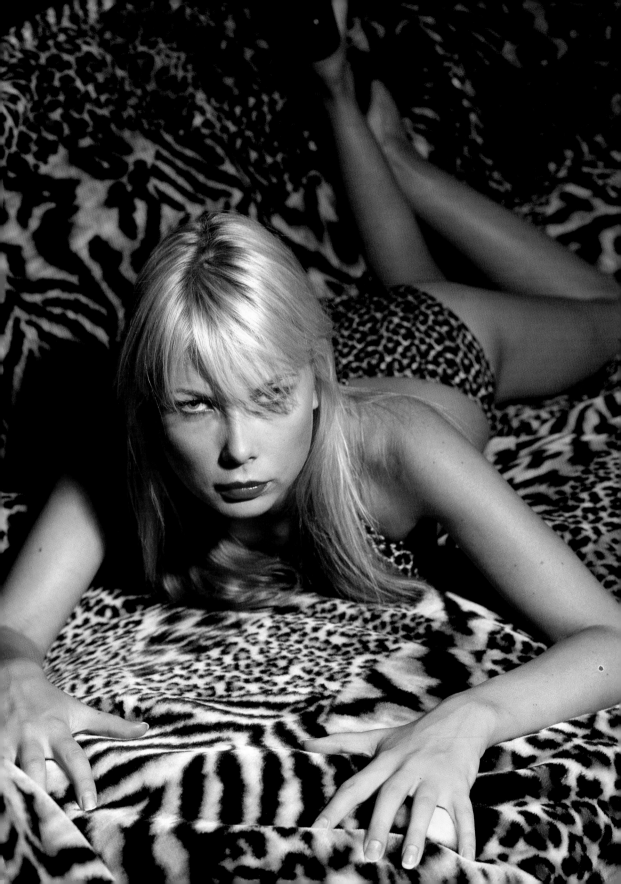

You won't be humiliatingly rejected, or discover that what's under those clothes isn't quite what you'd imagined *or* that the object of your desire gives the worst oral sex you've ever had (the ultimate sin). If you (like most people) struggle with balancing the pros of monogamy (history, soulmate connection, love, comfort, kids, support) with the cons (no new flesh to press, having to say no to constant temptation—just because you're in love doesn't mean you don't find others attractive), a rich fantasy life could offer the solution and keep everyone happy. Ninety-five percent of us have daily sexual fantasies—yes, even your granny, sitting there innocently knitting, could be ripping the shirt from that tasty gent who sits next to her at bingo *right this moment* (though let's not dwell on that one).

Don't edit the contents of **your own fantasies** in an effort to make them "normal." The whole point of a fantasy is to **escape from rule-bound, politically correct, desire-squashing social acceptability.**

YOUR OTHER LOVER

According to statistics, at some point 85 percent of people fantasize about someone else during sex with a partner—so there's no need to feel guilty about that either. While you're guiltily conjuring up Brad Pitt, oiled up and on his knees, he's transformed you into a Pamela Anderson balloon-breasted blonde with really tacky plexiglass heels. Does it mean you'd both seriously rather be with those people? Well... for a split second, probably yes. Would you do it in reality? Probably not—99 percent out of loyalty and 1 percent because the chance will never present itself (or have I got the statistics the wrong way around?). A fantasy is nothing but a capricious wish, and most experts dispel the idea that hot thoughts lead to betrayal—any sex therapist worth their salt will encourage you both to fantasize! In most cases, we have no intention or desire to play them out. Having a fantasy is not necessarily a form of planning ahead.

So why do we need to fantasize if we're getting good sex at home? Most evidence suggests that after the newness of a relationship wears off, most of our sexual turn-ons do not come from our partner. This doesn't have to be the case (and if you put this book to good use, I can pretty much

The single most potent engine driving sexual desire is our imagination. Fantasies are nature's built-in aphrodisiac for when your sex life gets off-track.

If your boyfriend's not well hung and you **tell him your fantasy about a guy with a 12-inch appendage**, the enthusiastic shine in your eyes will be met by an angry glint in his.

guarantee it won't be), but much of the passion we feel long-term, which leads us to want sex, is evoked by other people or situations. This does not—and I repeat, does not—mean you or your partner are going to be unfaithful in real life. It does mean, however, you're both unfaithful in your heads an average of 65,000 times per day (a slight exaggeration, perhaps, but you get my drift).

A VIBRATOR FOR THE MIND

When I was 20 and madly in love, I used to mercilessly quiz my then-fiancé: Did he lust after anyone else? Did he ever think about anyone else? Over and over again. The poor bastard. He used to reassure me constantly, "No, of course not. You're the only one I see, the only one I fantasize about, the only one I dream about." Twenty-three years later, I realize what a load of BS that was. The guy was normal! (I was normal, too, and having lots of fantasies about everyone and anyone, but, of course, applied the universal law that it was alright for me to do it, but not him.) Age and experience have taught me there are certain questions you shouldn't ask because your lover will

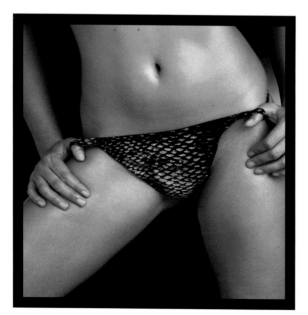

be forced to lie. And "Do you ever fantasize about anyone else?" is up there at the top of the list. If they don't, they're abnormal. Far from harming your sex life, your partner's fantasies about other people are helping it stay active. One study found people who fantasize during sex feel a greater level of sexual satisfaction and have fewer sexual problems, even if the fantasy figure is not their partner. Another study concluded that sexual fantasies help many married women achieve sexual arousal and/or orgasm during sex, irrespective of the quality of the love-making. Fantasies are nicknamed "a vibrator for the mind" for good reason: fantasizing during sex can mean the difference between OK sex and *fantastic* sex.

Women watch men the way men watch women: we also home in on the good parts. These images act as springboards for erotic daydreams.

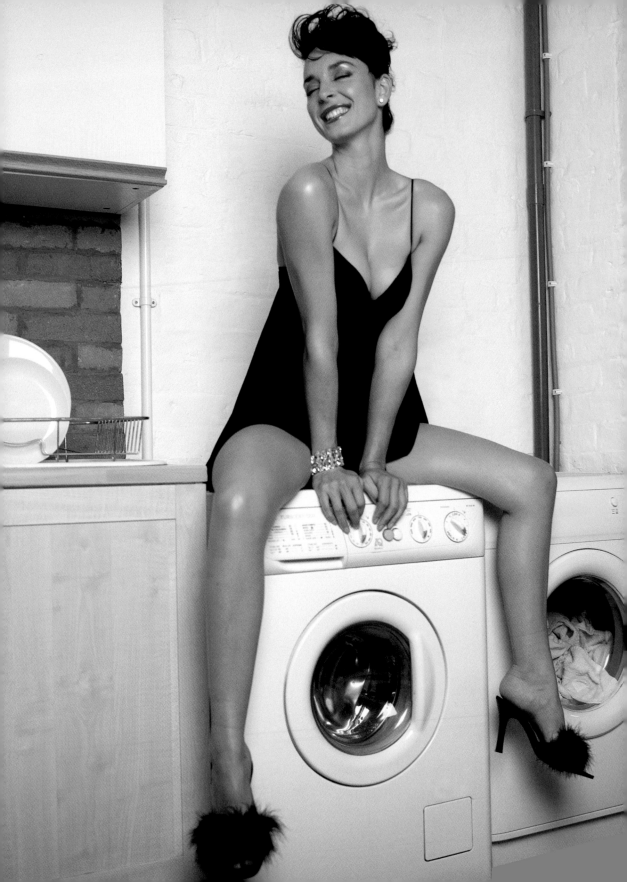

The obvious next question is this: if we all do it, and it's normal and even encouraged, why don't we all just confess our fantasies to our partners? Here's where expert opinion divides sharply. Some say yes, some say no. I straddle the fence. I think confessing some fantasies, after carefully thinking through the consequences (see pages 48–49), can be extremely exciting. But tact is imperative. If your boyfriend's not terribly well hung and you excitedly share a fantasy about sleeping with a guy with a 12-inch, rock-hard appendage, chances are the enthusiastic shine in your eyes will be met by an angry glint in his. Fantasies about anyone in real life—someone you work with, best friends, bosses, etc.—are threatening.

Fantasies might be common in humans, but there's another thing that is just as common: jealousy. Do you really want to know your husband spends hours dreaming about his colleague naked? No. Fantasies about celebrities are usually OK (presuming you're not dating one, with ready access to said celeb in the green room). As are situational fantasies that include your partner and no one else—though even they need to be thought through if they involve something like S & M or taking a different type of shower than the one offered in your bathroom.

DICEY OR JUST DARING

There's another reason why sharing fantasies often isn't necessary: they're private and sometimes evolve around thoughts we desperately, fervently hope our partner *never* guesses are whirling around in our head. Most of the fantasies most of us have, we'd never want to try in reality. So if you're worried your imagination is taking you to some decidedly dicey places to visit some rather seedy characters, don't worry. In almost all cases, a "weird" fantasy does not translate to your being a weirdo in real life. Just about all of us are drawn to the "dark side" of sexuality. We might wrinkle our noses at lap dancers and strippers, branding them "distasteful" when in polite company, but you can bet your next orgasm they've featured heavily in fantasy land. His are fueled by a sneaky real-life trip with the guys to see one, hers by a secret desire to be one and have all those men finding her completely irresistible...

Fantasies are the butter on the sliced bread of your sex life! So put the guilt trip to rest (if you're still suffering, turn to pages 60–61) and let's move onto some practical stuff: acting out a selected few, interpreting others, and finding how your partner's fantasies may differ very markedly from your own.

Can you reach orgasm simply by thinking about sex? Fantasy orgasm, first documented in 1992, proved the body's response to an imagery-induced orgasm was the same as one brought on by physical touch. Research is continuing, and neuropsychologists believe it could provide a solution for the 43 percent of women who are dissatisfied in bed. Further evidence that sexual arousal happens between the ears rather than the thighs!

Porn vs. plot
His and her sexual fantasies

Here's something that will surprise you (not): men's fantasies tend to resemble porn flicks—instant action, close-ups of bits sliding into bits, graphic detail, and a focus on the physical. Often they just need one simple image.

Men also tend to fantasize about women they've got a chance with in real life. Their leading ladies are approachable, girl-next-door types (though the odd celeb begging to be taken does pop up—or down, as the case may be). They're aware the chance of coming across a neighbor sunbathing topless, fingers playing along the edge of her bikini bottoms, is a tad more likely than a naked Angelina Jolie popping by. The higher the real-life probability, the more it arouses them. Whereas women, on the other hand, have no problems picturing George Clooney frothing at the mouth at the chance to slip a hand up their skirt.

Women's fantasies are based more around a situation: they set the scene (hunky repairman comes to door, etc.), then move on to specific sexual treats (oral sex featuring heavily). There's more conversation in women's fantasies as the narrative unfolds, whereas men tend to pepper theirs with grunts and groans of "oh, baby" and simple sentences like "look at my big **** disappearing into your little ****". Men say they think about things they've experienced, whereas women fantasize mainly about things they have never done. No prizes for guessing why this might be the case. It's more acceptable for men to experiment with the sordid side of sex than us "nice girls," so they've usually got a bigger base of experience to draw from. Men idealize themselves and their body parts (pecs and penises expand to enormous proportions); women might add the odd inch to an undersized chest and take some off other parts, but our idealizing is more likely to be done on the person we're pulling in the fantasy. It's no surprise that men fantasize more when they're not getting it, but what is interesting is that women do the opposite. We're more likely to work ourselves into a lascivious lather when we're having loads of good sex regularly. This supports a theory about female sexuality: without stimulation, our libido retreats into a slumber. Use it or lose it—literally.

He thinks *"I think most women would be totally shocked if they really knew what their partner fantasizes about—virtually everyone and everything. While we're making small talk with her friends from the office, we're mentally undressing every one of them, wondering what it would be like to have their mouths wrapped around our penis, what it would feel like to be inside them."*

The Top 20 Male Fantasies

- **Fantasies** about previous or anticipatory sex with a current partner.
- **A threesome**—usually watching two women having sex, then joining in. Great if it's sisters, heaven-sent if it's twins.
- **Sex with a woman** other than your partner (the ultimate: sex with a celeb in front of your friends).
- **Anonymous**, spontaneous sex with a stranger.
- **Group sex** with a multitude of gorgeous women lining up to give you oral sex.
- **Unending oral sex** dispensed by just about every female you come into contact with.
- **Anal sex.**
- **Secretly** watching a woman undress and masturbate.
- **Sex in a public** or risky place.
- **Being seduced** by an older woman.
- **Seducing** a virgin.
- **Spying** on two other people having sex.
- **Having sex** with your friend's girlfriend.
- **S & M**—being tied up and spanked or whipped.
- **Sex with forbidden people**—your girlfriend's mother, your boss.
- **Sex** with a sex worker.
- **Watching** your partner be taken by another man.
- **Sex** with another man.
- **Being watched** and applauded for your sexual expertise.
- **A "pretend"** rape scenario.

The Top 20 Female Fantasies

- **Fantasies** about previous or anticipatory sex with a current partner.
- **Sex with a man other than your partner**—seducing a friend or friend's partner is a favorite.
- **Sex** with a woman.
- **Sex** with someone at work.
- **A threesome** with two men, both fighting over your glorious body.
- **Sex** with a celebrity.
- **Being given expert oral sex**—under the desk at work, under the table at a restaurant.
- **Sex with a stranger**—with a penchant for repairmen when you're home alone.
- **Being found irresistible** (a line of male supermodels, especially the ones in the Calvin Klein ads, jostling to get to you).
- **Being a sex worker** (the ultimate "nice girl" sin).
- **Romantic fantasies**—hot sex in a magical location like a white, sandy beach.
- **Being deflowered** as a sacrificial virgin.
- **Being watched** with the voyeur desperate to trade places with the person you're having sex with.
- **Being forced to strip** in front of a crowd of men.
- **Playing Mrs. Robinson** and deflowering a male virgin.
- **Having an army** of physically perfect men as sex slaves.
- **Being "forced"** to have sex.
- **Starring in a porn film**—being lusted over worldwide.
- **Being seduced** by an authority figure.
- **S & M**—being tied up and spanked or whipped.

She thinks "Men have this skewed view that women's fantasies are all about handsome masked men, sidling up to us on the street to present us with a flower and an equally flowery speech about the color of our eyes. In reality, we dream up dirty, raw scenarios. The guy's more likely to rip our top open, roughly pull up our skirt, and perform hot oral sex with fingers in all orifices. And that's the mild version."

But what does it all mean?
An analysis of fantasies that leave us wondering

Interpreting fantasies is a bit like interpreting dreams—events and objects symbolize different things to different people. If you love the ocean, a dream of drifting aimlessly out to sea could represent freedom. If you get palpitations when dipping your toe in the pool, it's an anxiety dream, conjuring up terror rather than tranquil bliss. All our fantasies are individual but tend to have common themes. I asked a selection of men and women to submit their fantasies for interpretation and picked two typical examples, and one—incest—that's a little more unusual and may be a cause for concern.

THE FANTASY: *Watching a roommate have sex*

"My fantasy is partly based on something that happened. I came home late one night, a little drunk, and noticed my roommate's bedroom door was ajar and the light was on. I crept up to it and pushed it a little, expecting to find her in bed reading. Her boyfriend was away, so I knew she'd be alone. Except she wasn't alone at all. I saw her tied to the bed and a naked man on top of her. I stepped back but continued watching, initially, to be absolutely sure there wasn't anything bad going on. Then I recognized the guy as a colleague of Jayne's who she'd had her eye on... and continued to watch, even though she wasn't in danger.

I found it an incredible turn-on and went back to my room and masturbated. The next day, I felt guilty, but it still never fails to turn me on. Sometimes in the fantasy, they invite me to join them. In reality, I'm not attracted to my roommate—or the guy—so what's going on?"

Helen, 26, a journalist

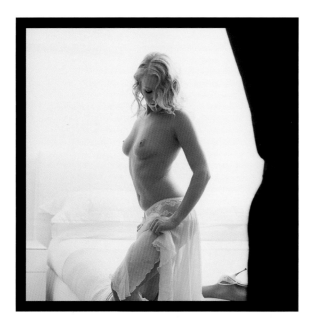

The analysis: Most people would be aroused in that situation, if they were honest! It's rare that we get the chance to watch real people have sex. It's even more fascinating watching one of our friends: you know her, but what's she *really* like? Is she a better lover than you are? Throw in the fact that it's not just forbidden to watch, but forbidden sex you're watching (she's cheating on her boyfriend) and you can see why Helen was turned on. The joining-in thing doesn't mean she's bisexual, just sexually curious. It also denotes sexual confidence: she secretly felt she could teach them both a thing or two!

She was putting on a show but, at the same time, seemed lost in her own private thoughts. It was unsettlingly erotic: was I in her head or was someone else?

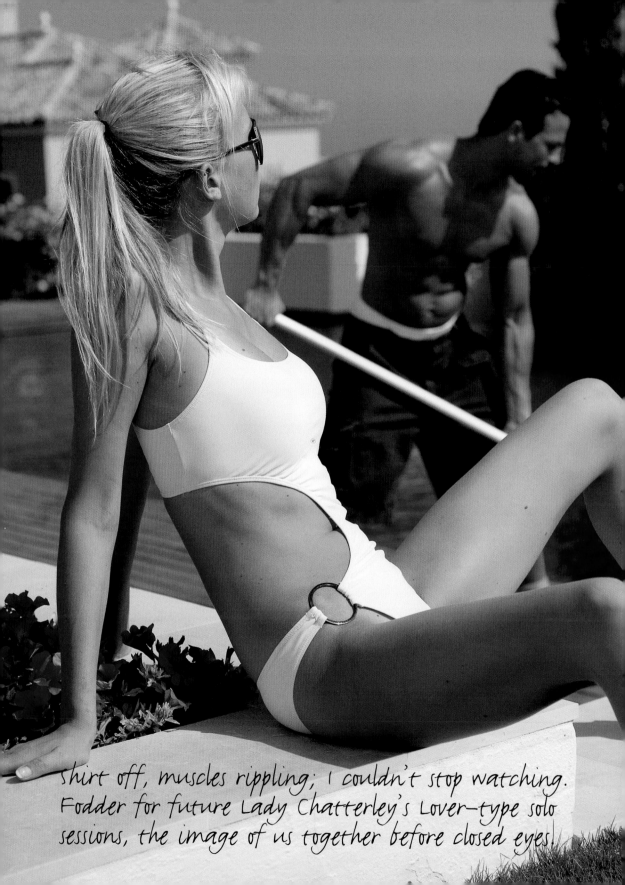

shirt off, muscles rippling; I couldn't stop watching.
Fodder for future Lady Chatterley's Lover-type solo
sessions, the image of us together before closed eyes.

THE FANTASY: *Sex with the same sex*

"I swear to God, I'm the straightest guy you'll ever meet, but I have a recurrent fantasy that scares the hell out of me. In it, I go to a gay club with my gay friends (I'm not homophobic, either) but instead of just hanging out with them, I go to the restroom and let a guy give me oral sex. I have no inclination to take it through to real life, but am I secretly gay? I don't think so, because I love having sex with women. I just don't understand why this gets me off."

Sean, 23, a student

Fantasies allow us the freedom to get sexually aroused by something without having to feel guilty or rejected afterward.

The analysis: I think this fantasy actually reflects a healthy attitude to sex. It doesn't mean Sean's gay: it just means he's bi-curious—a simple curiosity about what it would be like to make love to someone of the same sex. (We figure if someone's got what we've got, they must know how best to give us pleasure.) Having gay friends means he's been in an environment where men freely kiss and touch—enough on its own to spark sexual thoughts.

The fact that Sean is not homophobic and has great relationships with women also suggests he's not gay. It's interesting, though, that while most women who have same-sex fantasies do nothing to turn them into reality, men are more likely to do so. It's because they're used to being sexual initiators (and are more likely to find a gay man who'll take them up on an offer of no-strings sex). This doesn't mean all men or even lots of them act out their fantasies; most don't.

Most adolescent and teenage boys go through same-sex experimentation ("how far can you pee" competitions and group masturbation to see who can hit a target, etc.). Young girls kiss, cuddle, and do much more, so often it's now seen as completely commonplace. The overwhelming majority of people who experiment in this way end up exclusively hetero as adults. As adults, women continue to kiss, cuddle, and snuggle up—it's totally acceptable. Not so for men. The more taboo Sean makes the fantasy, the more arousing it will be. When he accepts that it's normal and nothing sinister, it will probably take its place as just one fantasy among many.

Adolescent same-sex experiences are significant. They're often our first sexual contact, and pleasurable, so they live on in fantasy land, even if we grow up to be heterosexual.

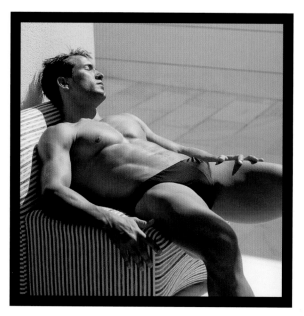

THE FANTASY: *Sex with a sibling*

"I used to masturbate to a fantasy about my brother. My father died when I was young and my brother assumed the 'head of the household' role and was always bossing me around. I resented it terribly, but one day, when I was masturbating, I conjured up a disturbing image of him coming into my room and telling me it was his job, as man of the house, to teach me about having sex with men. I resisted but he overpowered me, and the next thing I know I'm enjoying it and giving in. Over the years, the fantasy moved on to include oral sex, him tying me up, whatever. It made our relationship incredibly difficult. I was repulsed by him and resentful that he seemed to have 'taken over' my brain. I was so disturbed by it, I eventually went to see a counselor, who explained the reasons why it might be happening—none of which included me secretly lusting after him. I was so relieved and stopped fantasizing about it almost immediately. But it still bothers me a bit."

Emily, 34, a lawyer

The analysis: Of all the fantasies, those involving parents, brothers, or sisters cause us the most distress—yet it's a fantasy most people have at some time. Therapist Andrew Stanway says, "Whenever someone says they don't fantasize, I suspect I'm not far away from an incest fantasy"— such is our desperate concern, it can stop us from allowing ourselves to fantasize altogether! Yet when you consider we learn much about our relationships with the opposite sex by watching an opposite-sex parent or sibling, it stands to reason that our brains subconsciously cast them in the role of fantasy lover as well, as a way of safely testing our sexuality. Because incest is such a taboo in our society, once the thought's occurred to us to fantasize about such a terrible thing, it's almost impossible to let go. It's a bit like saying, "Don't think about pink elephants." That's all you'll then think about all day.

Well-meaning but inappropriate behavior from parents or siblings can also cause it. Most kids around three to five years old go through a stage of wanting to marry their opposite-sex parent (and wishing the same-sex one would disappear). It's a crucial stage of growing up: we're testing how important we really are—and the resulting lesson, that Mommy and Daddy can't be split up, teaches us about love triangles and that some people are unobtainable. If we do win Mommy's or Daddy's affections and attention, it can lead to confusion. If parents act more like partners, our subconscious starts to think of them in this way, and early fantasies are based on them. Other sibling fantasies may result from people questioning a close brother/sister relationship—snide comments about "you two being too close." The thought's abhorrent, but once suggested, "pink elephant syndrome" takes effect.

No that was real it was. My husband I thought I was looking at the view, and indeed I was. Such physical perfection. I want to touch him, see if he's real.

The confessions checklist
Crucial questions to consider

Sharing fantasies requires trust—it's not something I'd do with a new partner (unless it's a purely sexual relationship and the whole idea is to be as naughty as possible!). Unless you're 100 percent sure the information won't be used against you or repeated to others (and how can you be sure if you haven't known them long?), don't do it. It's a good idea to consider *all* of the following *before* opening your mouth, to make sure neither of you is in for any nasty surprises.

When and how are you going to confess the fantasy?

Choose your moment and mentally rehearse what you're going to say. If you feel uncomfortable saying it, close your eyes or look away, or consider writing it down. Never make a fantasy a complete surprise—what turns you on might leave your partner cold. Many a sitcom has got its loudest laughs from scenarios in which the housewife answers the door dressed as a nurse, to find her husband standing with his boss, brought home for dinner. It doesn't just happen in sitcoms.

Is your partner super-sensitive?

Some people react defensively to new sexual requests, taking it as a criticism that your current lovemaking isn't enough. If this is the case, use an indirect approach (see "Cunning ploys," opposite).

Will it make them jealous?

Any fantasies about real people you know or are likely to meet are out for obvious reasons. You can keep the sense of the fantasy, just make sure the person remains anonymous.

How out there is it?

If you've had your fantasy for a while, its initial shock value may have been diluted for you. Anything that involves sleeping with other people, "fake rape," some kind of swinging, or S & M could shock your partner initially, even if you have no desire to act it out. Start with "safe" scenarios.

What do you want to happen after you've confessed?

Why are you telling your partner? Do you want to take it through to reality? Are you asking them to join you or for their permission for you to indulge? Do you want to role-play it with them? Or are you just telling for a bit of sexy mood-setting? It's a *very* good idea to tell the person what you'd like to do with the fantasy *before* you tell them what it is.

What if they react badly?

If your partner appears to overreact to a mild fantasy, you may have hit a sensitive spot: it might remind them of a previous, traumatic experience. Stay calm and talk about the possible reasons why.

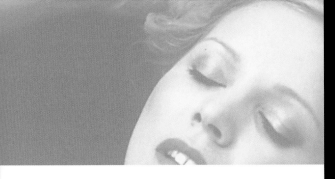

CUNNING PLOYS TO GET WHAT YOU WANT
(without having to ask outright)

If you're not the type to say, "Honey, let's skip the dishes and instead you pop on a pair of my lace panties, pretend you're a female sex worker, and let me seduce you?", you might find the following useful. There are ways to bring up a fantasy you'd like to role-play, without having to ask cold—or risk embarrassment. Pick the category you fall into, then white-lie your way into the lustiest sex you've had in ages...

You're nervous about their reaction: Wait until you're both in a jovial mood, then say you had an erotic dream. Tell them about it (a made-up scenario based around your fantasy) and see what reaction you get. The more detail they ask for, the more interested they are. Take that as your cue to confess it's been a fantasy of yours for ages. Keep the conversation light-hearted, then ask about their fantasies. Once you're both talking, it's relatively easy to suggest acting them out for a bit of fun.

You're not sure about their reaction: Rent a movie with a scene that features or resembles your fantasy. Watch their face as it's playing: are they intrigued or horrified? If they're watching avidly, snuggle up sexily and say "God, how hot is this!". Then move in for the kill ("Hey, I've got a great idea", etc.).

You're reasonably confident they'll go for it: Buy your lover a sex book based on or including your fantasy theme as a present. If they're shy, let them read it alone first before asking which were their favorite bits. If they're secure sexually, put Post-it notes throughout the book on pages or pictures that particularly appeal to you, before wrapping it up.

Toxic turn-offs:

- **Punishing your partner for suggestin[g] you try something new:** Remember, people need variety to stay interested. It doesn't mean your partner is tired of you, just that they want a new experience.

- **Refusing to try something reasonabl[e]** If it won't harm you, try not to say no just because you think you won't like it. How do you know if you've never tried it?

- **Making veiled threats to leave or get "it" elsewhere if they don't comply:** If your partner won't be persuaded, either accept defeat graciously and suggest an alternative (recommended); do it with someone else (dicey at best); or, if you thi[nk] you can't be true to yourself unless you ha[ve] this experience regularly end your existing relationship and find someone who wants [to do] what you do (sometimes necessary).

Works every time

- **Suggesting an alternative:** If his reque[st] to watch you mud-wresting your best frien[d] naked, doesn't appeal, just say no... but m[ake] it clear you're open to other suggestions.

- **Trying something that doesn't appea[l] to you at least once:** Lots of people fin[d] role-play embarrassing but then enjoy som[e] aspects of it (e.g., spanking, being tied up).

- **Respecting not everyone has the sam[e] desires:** You don't expect to be clones in [all] other areas of your life, so why the bedro[om]

Sharing sexy stuff
How to get a fantasy from your head, into your bed

We'd rather die than try some fantasies in reality. But others... well, you might not want to replicate them exactly, but you'd sure as hell like to capture the tummy-aching, skin-tingling, vagina-moistening, penis-lifting effect it has on your libido! Role-playing fantasies is one way to get the kick—without any of the malevolent misfires sometimes experienced by taking them through to real life. Here you'll find tips, hints, and example scenarios to help you turn erotic thoughts into sexy, real-life escapades.

ex play is like any other game—except there **e** no losers. **You both win with bigger, etter, raunchier orgasms!**

ROLE-PLAY RULES
As with every game, following a few basic guidelines will make everything run much more smoothly.

- **It doesn't have to be a literal translation**—symbolism is often all that's needed. Got a threesome fantasy? Describing what could be happening if two men were there could give a sense of having two men doing different things simultaneously.
- **Expensive props** aren't necessary, but the more effort you make, the better it usually is. Use music and different rooms of your house for different scenarios.
- **Try to choose fantasies** that appeal to both of you, particularly the first time around.
- **Work out the scenario together** beforehand: often, that's just as much of a turn-on as acting it out.
- **Be specific about** how "in character" you want each other to be—for some people, slipping back into your usual selves, even for a minute, destroys the illusion.
- **Don't worry if you laugh**—just keep going. Lust will usually overtake the laughter once you start getting into it.
- **Work out an agreed "stop now" signal** in case you don't like it as much as you thought! Make your "stop" word something that isn't ever going to be used as part of the role-play. "Purple" is better than "more" for obvious reasons.

Tailor the fantasy to her personality. She's girly and giggly? Try silk stockings and gentle threats. Ballsy, cigar-smoking types go for handcuffs and barked commands.

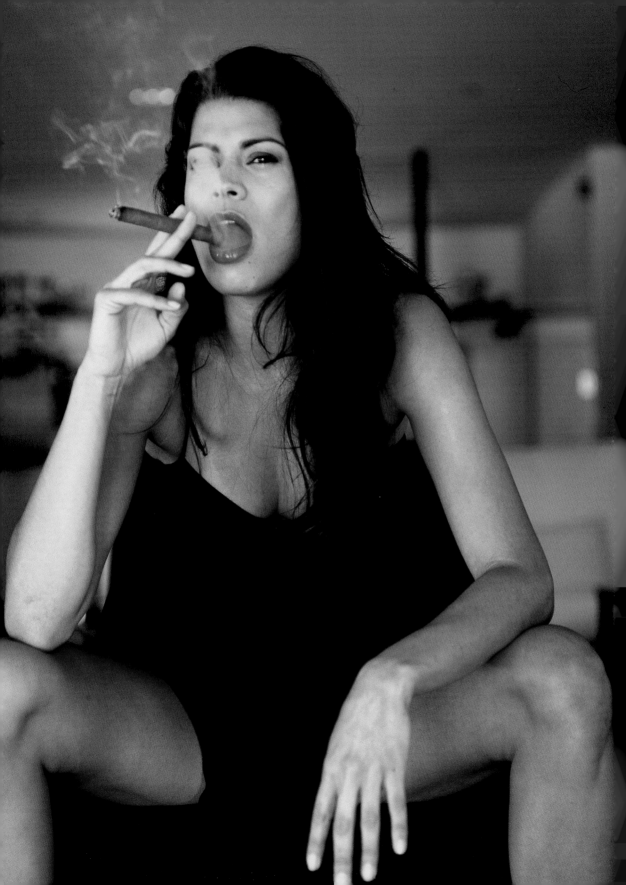

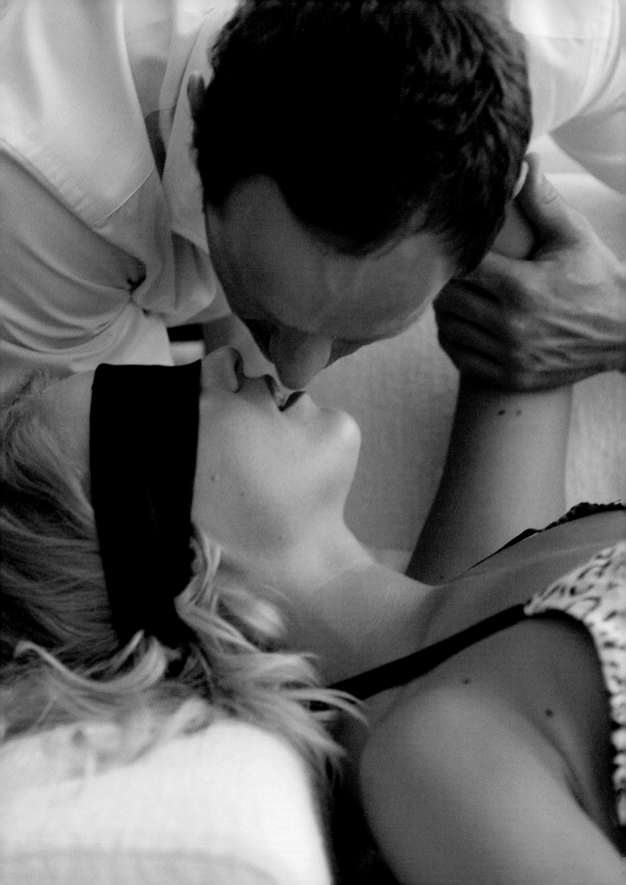

- **Choose your time** and place to act out the fantasy: no roommates, dogs begging for walks, children wanting to know where their Batman suit disappeared to.
- **Don't be scared** to start the fantasy in public. Some—like "sex with a stranger"—lend themselves to the two of you meeting up in a bar before the real action starts. As long as you don't dress weirdly or act abnormally, no one ever needs to know.

Blindfolds mean they can **feel, smell,** and **taste** you, but not see what's happening. **Each touch, kiss, lick** is loaded with **sensory surprise.**

LET THE GAMES BEGIN...

These are two popular role-play scenarios to help you bring your fantasies to life. Feel free to add your own twists and surprises along the way...

THE FANTASY: Deflowering a "virgin"

Why it appeals: It's a power game with both submissive and dominant roles, each with its pluses. Men particularly like playing the virgin, after a lifetime of being the sexual persuader.

What you'll need: If she's doing the seducing, a "sexy secretary" outfit works well: a long pencil skirt, shirt unbuttoned to show off a push-up bra, stockings, high heels. Think Mrs. Robinson.

The action plan (her seducing him):

- Get both of you a drink, then take him into the lounge. He sits on the couch, you sit opposite, crossing your legs and hiking your skirt up. He's not sure where to look.
- Make chit-chat to suit the scenario (he's your friend's son who's dropped in to mow the lawn, or the shy pizza delivery boy), then make it saucier. Tell him you don't think your husband finds you attractive. Does he think you're attractive? What parts? Why? Let him squirm as he tries to be politically correct—and hide the erection that is starting to happen. At which point you say...
- "You're looking a little uncomfortable. Let me help you." And you move from the chair to sit beside him on the couch.

Women who rate themselves as good lovers fantasize frequently. And if you prepare for future sex through anticipatory fantasies, you're likely to be more easily aroused and enjoy sex more when it happens. Fantasies are just the thing to transform you from tired commuter or worn-out mom to sultry sex goddess. The right scenario played in your head could be just what you need to push you over the brink from uninterested to erotically charged.

- You loosen the first two buttons of his shirt, telling him he looks hot and bothered. Rub your hand against his exposed chest, saying, "Such soft skin. So different from my husband's... ".

- As he squirms, you undo the top few buttons of your shirt, take his hand, and place it on the underside of your breast. Ask him what it feels like and if he likes the feeling. Keep making small talk. Ask him if he's ever made love to a woman before. He'll squeak out, "No." Ask him if he'd like to make love to you... It's OK, you won't tell and no one's going to walk in.

- Ask him to take off your top and your bra. Tell him to touch your breasts and instruct him on how to do it. Moan and sigh, but you're still the grown-up, so don't get too out of control.

- Ask him to stand up in front of you, unzip his pants, and take out his (by now) throbbing penis. Admire it, say how hard it is compared to men your age, then give him exquisitely torturous oral sex—stopping just short of orgasm. The idea is to bring him to a tantalizing peak but not to the point of ejaculatory inevitability (when a dozen vestal virgins couldn't stop him from climaxing).

- Undress yourself—theatrically and maintaining eye contact throughout. Let his eyes caress your body, but don't let him touch you. Leave on your high heels, stockings, and garter belt. Pose provocatively, caress your curves. Ask him if he likes what he sees and if he wants to touch you.

- Undress him, then lead him to the bed and promise to explain how to make love to a woman to make her scream. Honor the promise. Each touch, kiss, fondle, thrust is his very first, remember.

sexual desire can be wickedly fueled by frustration. She's naked, he's allowed to watch but not touch; she can have oral sex but must not orgasm.

At first he touches reverently, then he's lost in a frenzy of passion.

- The fantasy ends when he loses control completely—which he will in about three minutes if you've played your part properly!

Some classic fantasy scenarios to whet your appetite...

- boss and secretary • burglar surprises sleeping beauty • biker gang "forces" innocent girl into doing naughty things • cheerleader and football team • doctor and nurse • firefighter rescues very grateful victim • prostitute and john • police arrest (complete with cuffs) • priest and nun • rock star and groupie • principal/teacher with student

THE FANTASY: The sex slave

Why it appeals: Having someone under our complete sexual command has obvious benefits. You don't have to worry about the "no, you first, honey" niceties of sex: it's all about YOUR pleasure. Meanwhile, the "slave" is "forced" to perform acts they'd secretly love to try, but wouldn't dare suggest.

What you'll need to act it out:

For this example, she's the slave and he's the master. Jeans and a leather jacket, undone over

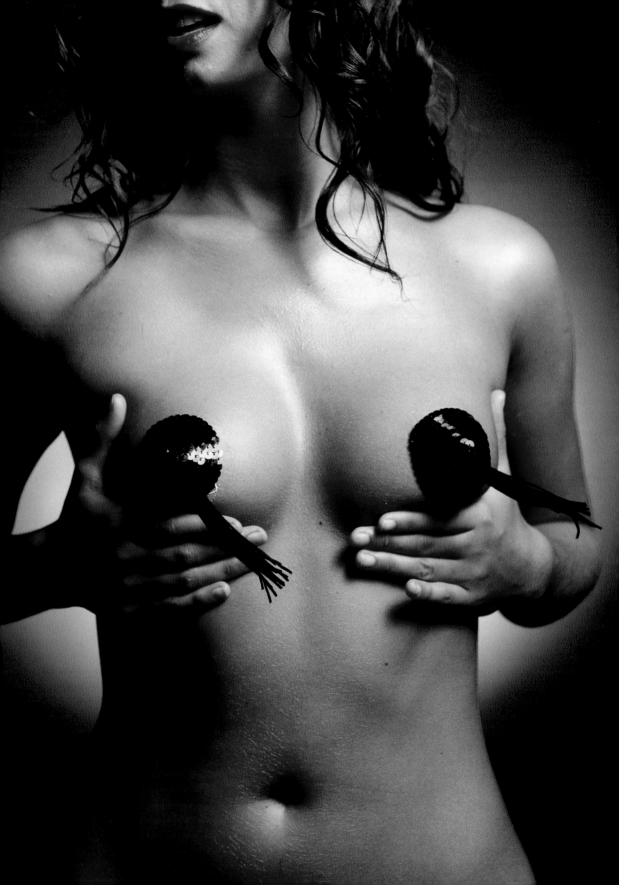

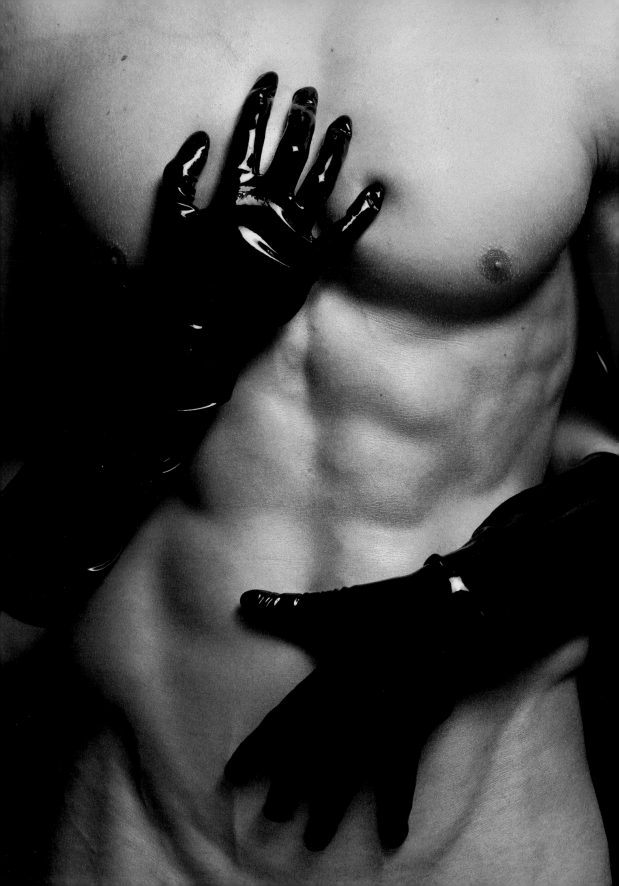

a naked chest, sets the scene nicely. You'll also need a blindfold, scarves or old stockings to tie her up, and a wooden spoon or hairbrush. She's completely naked—helpless and vulnerable (exactly how you want her!).

Don't assume that **what did the trick** the night before will **put a twinkle in their eye** the next day. Our moods and **desires** change constantly.

The action plan:

- Try to keep an expressionless face. Don't say, "Are you OK?", "Did I hurt you?", "Are you sure you're enjoying this?" This isn't about her, it's all about you!!! You're the master, she's the slave!
- Start by ordering her to do small tasks—get you a drink, fluff up the pillows, give you a massage.
- Don't ask, order. Make it clear you are the boss and she is not to misbehave or she'll be punished (spank her with the wooden spoon or back of the hairbrush).
- Once you're both nicely in character, order her to sit or lie down, face turned away from you, blindfold her, and tie her hands behind her back. Push her forward into a submissive position. She's now naked, bound, and blindfolded—completely at your mercy!
- Grab your wooden spoon or brush and administer a few short, sharp whacks on her bottom— even better if she begs you to stop.
- Start caressing her. Reach in between her legs— wait until she's moaning for more, then stop.
- Tell her you decide what she gets and when—and she has to satisfy you first.
- Turn her around and order her to pleasure you. She can use her mouth; untie her hands if you want, but keep the blindfold on.
- No matter how pleasurable, punctuate her stimulation of you by pushing her away when she seems to be enjoying herself the most. Tell her she's been a bad girl.
- Tease her: start to give her oral sex, then stop. Push your fingers inside her and when she starts thrusting against them, stop.
- The fantasy ends by you announcing (dramatically) that she's now free from her slavery—to service you.

Sexual fantasies usually revolve around control, and the amount of power the person has in real life often dictates how much they want in their fantasy life. After a day of being the top decision-maker, being bossed around in the bedroom could be a CEO's idea of power paradise. Someone who's bullied relentlessly by superiors will usually opt for a rapturous role reversal where they get to wield the whip (perhaps literally).

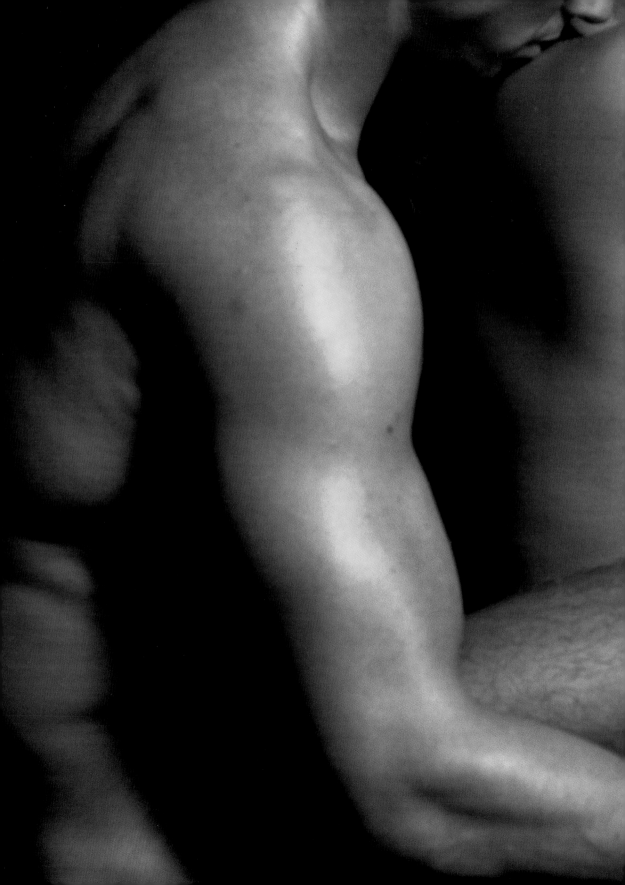

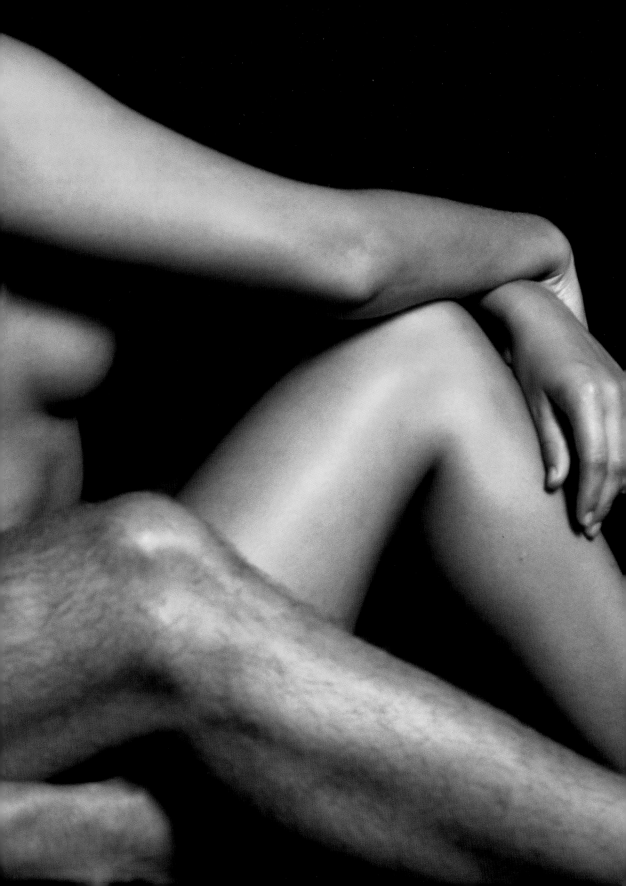

Guilty pleasures
(Seriously, do you think I'm weird for thinking that?)

Now here's a comforting thought: no one has figured out how to read minds yet. Which means it doesn't really matter what filthy thoughts are floating around in there!

If you choose, no one but you need know about your fantasies. If they bring you pleasure, cause no one else pain, and worry you simply because they're a little politically incorrect or "weird," my advice would be to give yourself permission to go for it! Still concerned? Then keep reading...

What if I don't like a fantasy and want it to stop?

Our fantasies, like the rest of our lives, are influenced heavily by what's happened to us. It's a lucky person who sails through without negative experiences, and these creep into our sexual scripts. Often, simply understanding where an urge comes from can stop you from worrying. (An upsetting spanking at school might cause you to fantasize about it later, for instance.) But if the remorse and confusion post-fantasy outweighs the pleasure you get during it, you can actively banish it. If you're masturbating and the fantasy pops into your head, stop and consciously think of something else that doesn't cause you angst. Replace old fantasies with new ones by masturbating while reading and watching erotica. During sex, focus on the here and now: how your lover's touch feels. If it helps, tell them how wonderful what they're doing feels. It's like breaking any other habit—you need to retrain your brain. Keep at it for a while and it should naturally slip away. If it doesn't and you're still worried, consider seeking professional help.

Am I weird if my fantasy is weird?

We'll often fantasize about things contrary to our core personality (Ms. Goody Two-Shoes becomes the star of a particularly dirty orgy) simply because they revolve around something we wouldn't dare do in real life. There is no evidence at all to support that simply fantasizing about something leads you to act

Finish the fantasy... You've checked in to a nice hotel and discover that it has erotic films. This makes you feel decidedly sexy, so you call for a massage. You take a bath and put on a robe over your naked body, and there's a knock at the door. You forget the film is playing, and as the man is setting up the table, you see him stealing glances at the screen. You lie down and he says, "Exactly what sort of massage would you like?"...

on it. Deviant fantasies can be an indicator of true sexual deviancy, but it's invariably coupled with real-life symptoms as well. So long as you can distinguish between fantasy and reality, it's not a fixation (see below), and you've got no desire to take it through to real life, there isn't usually a problem.

What if I don't have fantasies?

Some people are great cooks, others can't quite get the hang of the toaster. Same deal here. Creative people conjure up vivid, technicolor fantasies with intricate plot twists, scene changes, and mood-lighting tweaks. Others have problems imagining themselves walking across a room. If you're the latter, try focusing on your favorite erotic scene from a movie or book, then individualize it. Put yourself in the lead role. Change it to suit you. Train yourself to pay attention to any sexy thoughts. Write them down, look for a theme, then think up a simple storyline based around that. See "Finish the fantasy" (below) for inspiration and, remember, a fantasy can be one simple image. It's also not compulsory to have them, by the way. If it doesn't do much for you, so be it. Some people adore poring over vacation brochures, making endless plans about what they'll do when they get there. Others buy tickets at the last minute, throw a T-shirt and sunscreen into a bag, show up, and see where it takes them. There's no right or wrong.

What if I fantasize too much?

It's a bit like asking if you masturbate too much. Assuming you're not interrupting an important meeting to relieve yourself in the washroom, your genitals aren't decreasing in size from too much rubbing, and you're able to watch a whole DVD without putting it on pause (and I'm talking Disney, not *Debbie Does...*), there is no such thing. If your fantasies aren't hurting anyone and you just have an active imagination, imagine away! Fantasizing keeps you on sexual simmer, which means your libido is alive and ready for action. How can that be bad? But if you only get aroused and orgasm by focusing on one particular fantasy, you could be heading for problems. It's the head equivalent of a fetish—when a person needs a particular object (like a lover wearing high heels) to achieve sexual satisfaction. Warning signs are needing, rather than wanting, the fantasy to arouse you, being more interested in the fantasy than your lover, or if your lover complains of you feeling detached or unconnected during sex. If this is happening, seek professional advice.

You're in an empty train car. An attractive girl gets on and sits across from you. She smiles but doesn't speak, just pulls out a book that, judging by the cover, is an erotic novel. As she reads, she steals glances at you, then rearranges herself so her skirt hikes up. She sees you watching and deliberately exposes more flesh. You take a chance, and put a tentative hand on the inside of her knee. She parts her legs, giving you permission to proceed...

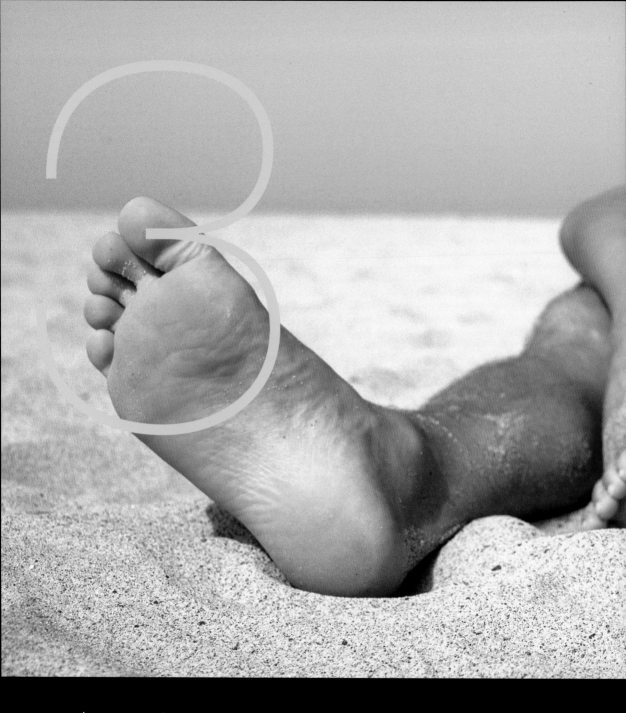

3

The quickest way to dust off and spark up a musty sex life? Take sex out of the bedroom and head outside for a risqué romp!

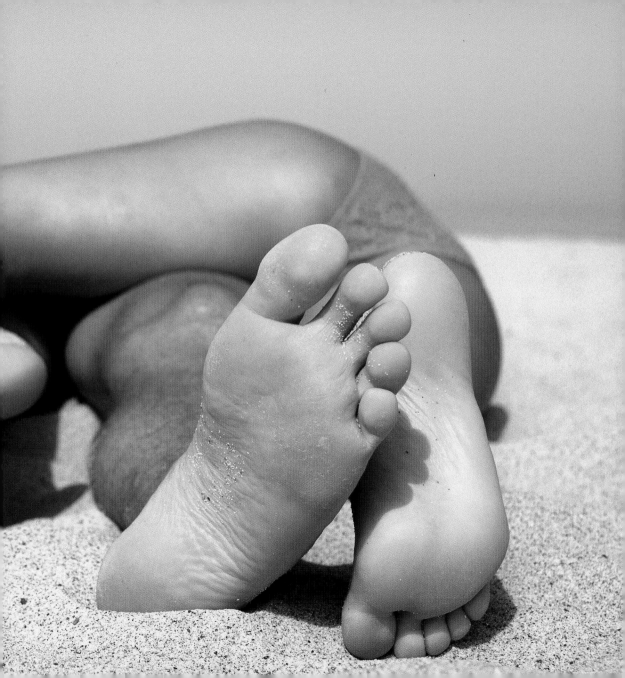

turn up the heat

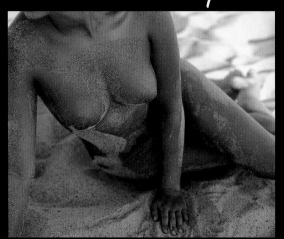

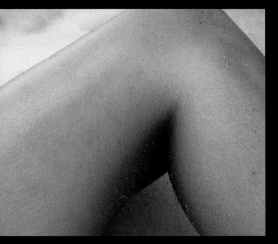

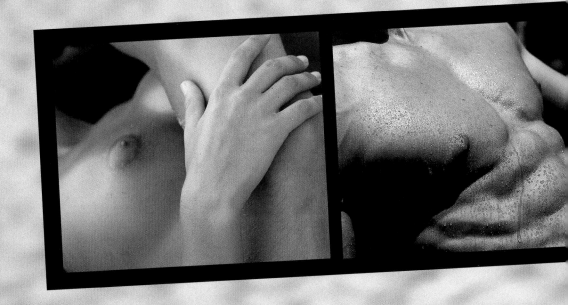

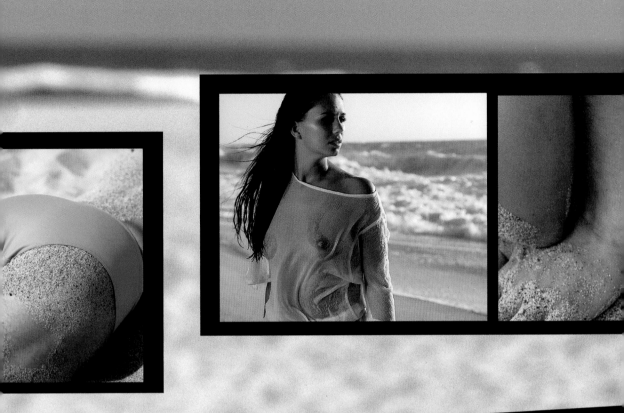

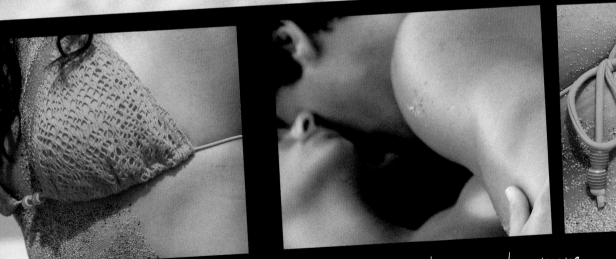

summer: we wear less, work less, drink more, play more— and think about sex almost as often as we breathe.

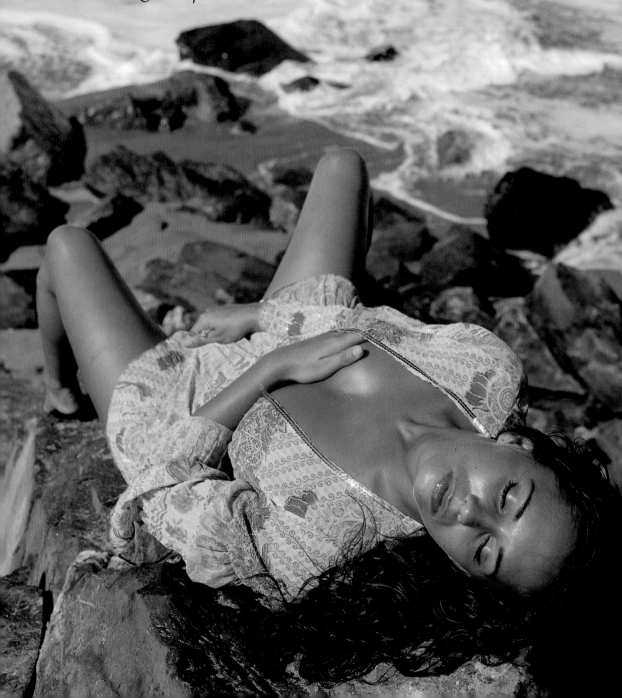

The sun makes you feel lazy and languid, the rhythmic pounding of the sea does the opposite, sparking lively fantasies of a sexy stranger who finds you sprawled on the rocks alone...

Sex and the great outdoors
How to make love in public *without* getting arrested

Breathe some fresh air into your love life—literally. The fear of discovery, pounding heartbeats, that delicious jolt of adrenaline when you think someone's coming (and it's not either of you two). Anyone who's ever had sex outside knows just how fantastic it can be. And as for that pesky problem of its being illegal to have sex in public (if you're caught and reported, you could go to jail), there are ways to indulge in alfresco sex discreetly. It's called being sensible. Assess each situation carefully, stay fully clothed (well, as much as possible), and use props to hide behind. A picnic blanket, sarong, or beach umbrella can disguise a multitude of naughty acts; if you're *really* shy, try a tent! It provides the privacy you need but still *feels* as though you're on display. Give one (or all) of the following a whirl...

Sex in a tent is legal—you're not in public view. But **"doing it"** as you hear others walking past, dangerously close, **feels wonderfully wicked.**

ON OR IN THE CAR
How you do it: Yes, you *could* slip into the backseat and enjoy relative privacy, but it's far, far, far sexier to do it on the car hood. She sits on the hood and he stands in front of her. She then wraps her legs around his waist to let him penetrate, then leans back on the hood, balancing herself with her arms. One word of caution, though, before you eagerly jump on board: the hood is made of metal. If you've been driving for a long time, it could be bottom-burningly *hot*. If you've been parked for a while and it's winter, it'll turn your cheeks to ice. Warm up the engine for five minutes or put a coat down to lean back on.

Why you'd risk it: It's uber-erotic because not only do you risk getting caught, it's the sort of thing teenagers do. You both recapture the heady thrill of adolescence, feeling wild, free, and terribly *un*grown-up.

Chances of getting caught: Choose a suitably quiet street or country road and the chances are low. Besides, you've got your getaway right there. If a car appears from nowhere, both drop down and pretend to be examining a flat tire.

"When you're choosing between two evils, always try to choose the one you haven't tried before."

Mae West

ON TOP OF A PICNIC TABLE

How you do it: Head to the park just at dusk, when everyone else (especially families) is leaving to go home. Pack supper, find a sturdy table provided in the picnic area, have a feast, then clear the table and devour each other! It's easy to accomplish this one: she lays back on the table and wraps her legs around his waist with him standing in front of her. This position works because she's facing one way, he's facing the other, so you can keep an eye out for intruders in each direction! If you can't find a table, have sex spoon-style (he penetrates from behind) while wrapped in the picnic blanket.

It's **raw sex at its best**, but not the best way to try out that new extend-an-**orgasm** technique. The problem with **standing positions** is that his **penis** isn't the only thing that gets stiff...

Why you'd risk it: I'm not a huge believer in all the supposed "hot spots" that continue to be "discovered" on the female body. On the other hand, anything that inspires you to try something new is fine by me! The picnic-table position is ideal for stimulating the supposed A-spot: the anterior fornex erogenous, which is just above the cervix at the innermost point of the vagina. In 1996, scientists "accidentally" hit on this hot spot while trying to find a cure for vaginal dryness. During their research, they found that 95 percent of women were massively aroused when this area was stimulated. Nearly all the female participants said it led to more intense and frequent climaxes, and many women had their first orgasm! The research methods that produced this astonishing result have since been questioned, but there's no harm in mounting a little expedition anyway!

Chances of getting caught: High. There's also no mistaking what you're up to if someone does stumble upon you, and picnic tables tend to be found in reasonably public areas, rather than in secluded countryside. Attempt under cover of darkness only in a secluded park.

Low-risk public sex venues:
- Relatively quiet public restrooms (and lots of them so people aren't kept waiting) with locks on the doors.
- Your backyard.
- A public park at night under a blanket.
- In the car in a parking ramp that isn't regularly patrolled.
- A rooftop.
- On a boat.
- The balcony of a hotel.
- A little-used stairwell.

UP AGAINST A TREE

How you do it: She stands, leaning back against a tree, and he stands in front of her. She then puts her arms around his neck and wraps

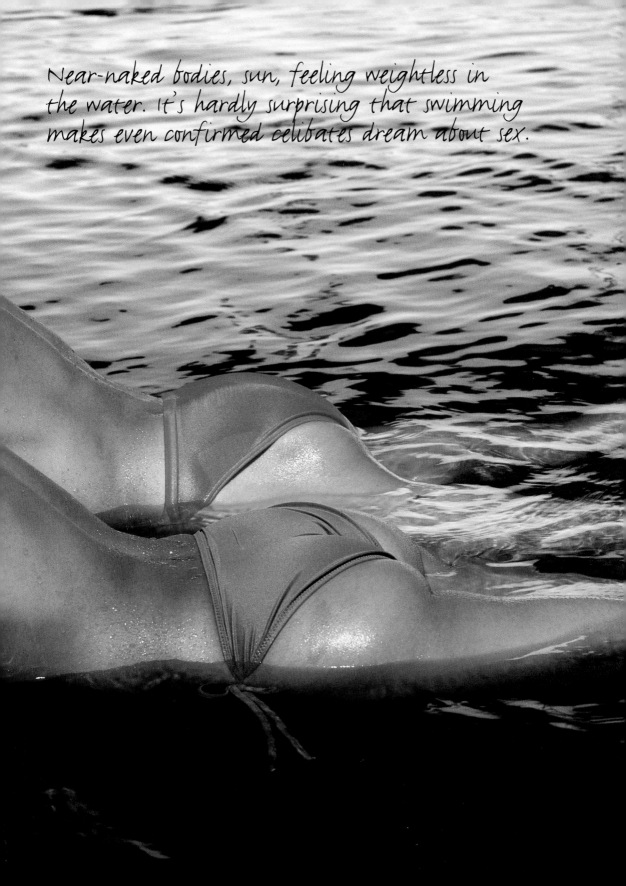

Near-naked bodies, sun, feeling weightless in the water. It's hardly surprising that swimming makes even confirmed celibates dream about sex.

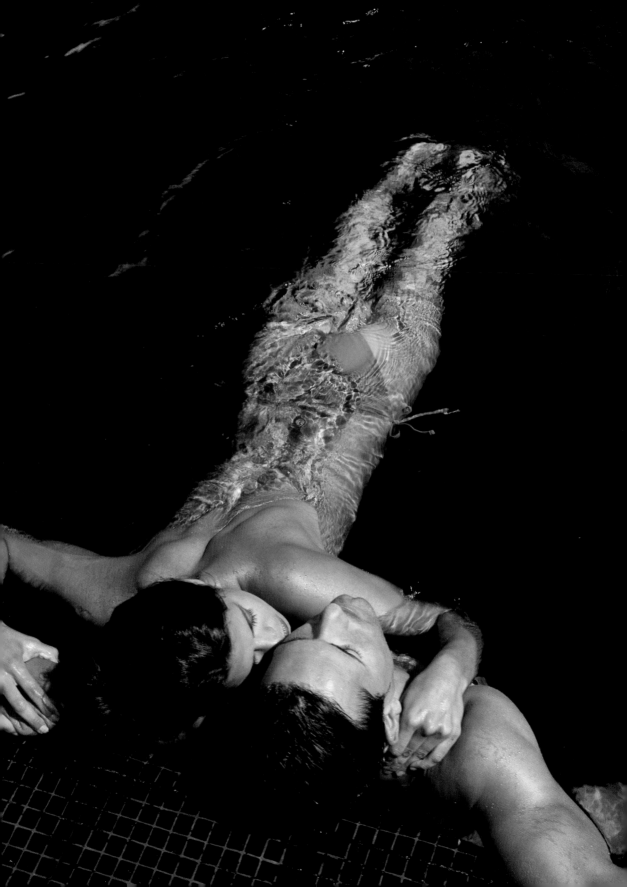

Forget winning the lottery. Recent studies show more and better sex with your partner, rather than lots of money, is what will make you happier.

her legs around his waist. For balance and support, she keeps her back firmly pressed against the tree and hangs onto any strong-looking branches. If that all sounds far too energetic, cheat! Get her to wrap one leg around his waist and keep the other on the floor. He should hold onto her thigh/s.

Why you'd risk it: Penetration is deep, snug, and tight because most of her weight is bearing down on his penis and her vagina is angled. If she squeezes her thigh muscles, she gives him super-tight friction. It's primal sex at its very best but still probably not the position to try out that new extend-an-orgasm technique. Standing positions tend to work only for quickies because his penis isn't the only thing that gets stiff.

Chances of getting caught: The bigger the woods, the more chance you have of finding a tree that is isolated. Keep an ear out for the telltale snapping of twigs (someone walking the dog) and it's not too difficult to untwine, fix your clothes, and pretend you're having an innocent smooch. Okay, they might make a big swerve around you, sniff disapprovingly, or look embarrassed, but they're only jealous!

ON A SWING

How you do it: If she's a good (naughty) girl, she'll have thought to wear a long, loose skirt and no panties. She lifts the skirt and sits forward on the seat. He stands in front, feet squarely placed on the floor, holds the sides of the seat firmly, and draws her to him to penetrate. It's then simply a matter of his swinging her back and forth while he remains standing still.

Why you'd risk it: It's fun! You're bound to end up laughing, reminding yourselves of the fun you used to have as a kid. Chances are you won't achieve deep penetration because of the difficulty in coordination, but that's not a bad thing. All of the nerve endings—or sensory receptors—in the vagina are located within an inch or so of the vaginal entrance.

Chances of getting caught: You may get away with it in a playground late at night, but—and it's a BIG but—if you get caught and reported, you'll risk arrest for being way too adult in a children's zone. Playgrounds are often in residential areas. If the neighbors might be suspicious if you install a swing in the garden, consider buying a sex swing that you suspend from the ceiling indoors.

Sex outside—the rules:
- Dress for sex (floaty skirts, no underwear, zip rather than button flies, uncomplicated bras).
- Avoid arrest by being aware of the laws in the country you're in.
- Have a code word or look that alerts you both to opportunities.
- Forget foreplay and instead use lube.
- Plan your escape and what to say if you get caught.
- Don't do it if being caught would be a nightmare.

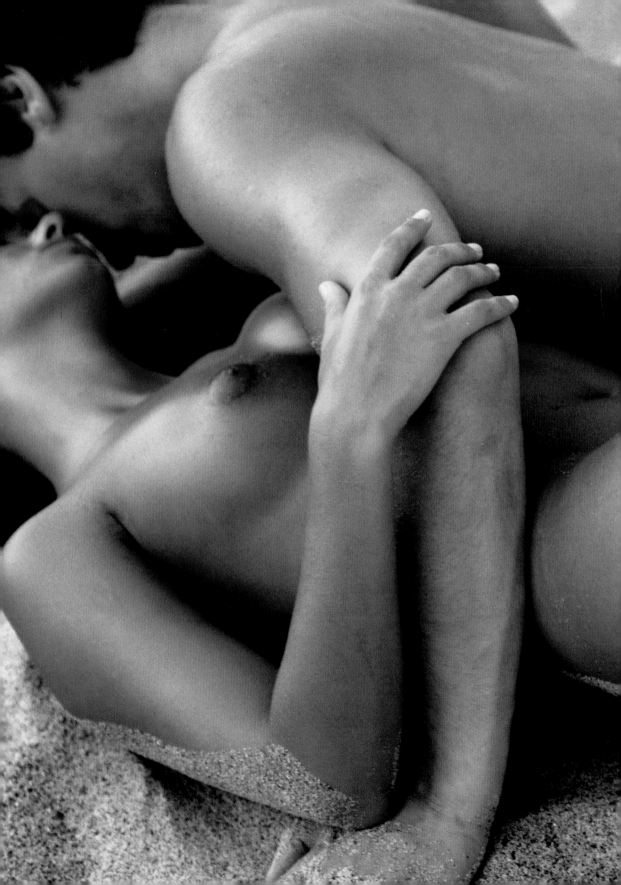

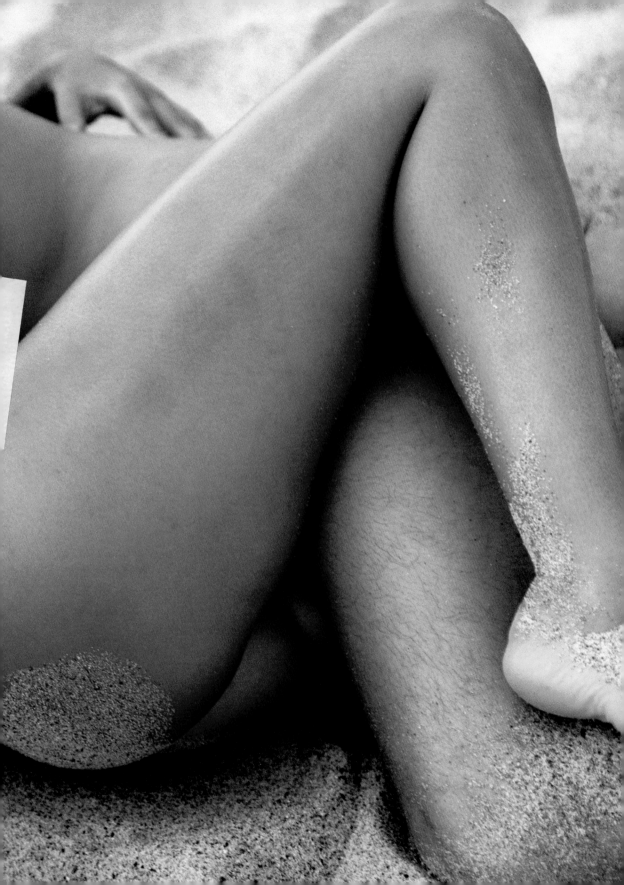

Outdoor sex... indoors
For those who don't dare do it alfresco

Some people are out the door with half their clothes ripped off the second you suggest having sex outside. Others aren't quite so adventurous. While you're revelling in the might-get-caught, rough-and-readiness of sex alfresco, they're peering worriedly over your shoulder, rather than gazing lustily at your breasts. Then there are the "Princess and the Pea" types—a pebble the size of a pinhead pricks their bottom, or it's one degree below balmy and the whole thing's ruined. And yes, I am speaking from experience.

"Let's do it right here, right now," I said to my new (sort-of) boyfriend, Richard. "What, here?" he said, looking around him with disbelief, as though we were standing in the middle of a department store during the after-Christmas sale and I'd suggested a bit of hanky-panky in the clearance aisle. We were, in fact, sitting at a picnic table near a river in pitch-darkness at midnight, a good five-minute walk from the dreadful resort (his choice) we were staying in. Since it was populated by people who took their teeth out and removed limbs at night, I dare say we'd have had time to get ourselves together even if we did hear an aluminum walker moving stealthily down the path.

To be fair, I may have sounded less than enthusiastic: it was a last-ditch attempt to save a struggling relationship, rather than a spontaneous impulse inspired by lust. The man I initially thought had high standards turned out to be persnickety. Who, on a supposed "dirty weekend," folds their underpants, color-codes their socks, and arranges their products with labels lined up on the shelf in the bathroom? (Who, while we're at it, takes back empty glass bottles and asks for the 5-cent deposit?) "What's wrong with having sex here?" I repeated defensively. "It's dirty!" he said, horrified. "And the table's hard and what are those white splats on it? And if you're thinking of doing it on the ground, well, that's wet and cold and awful. Is that what you were thinking of?" he said, fixing me with an "I *knew* you were weird" stare.

If you're dating a Richard (please tell me you haven't married one!) or linked up with a nervous Nellie, it still doesn't mean you have to miss out on the excitement of sex outside. Simply recreate the urgency of fast, furious, have-to-hurry sex by indulging in a few inventive indoor quickies. Adding some quick sex sessions into the mix is a great way to improve your sex life generally. Quick sex is better than no sex—and that's often what happens with busy couples. Quickies keep you connected as a couple and ensure that your appetite for sex stays high. Here's how:

DO IT IN DIFFERENT PLACES

A quickie in bed, where you always have sex, doesn't quite have the exotic flavor you're after. It needs to be somewhere unorthodox, where you haven't ever (or don't usually) have sex. Try any of the following and, to make it really interesting, put a time limit on it. No more than five minutes from start to finish—and remember, a quickie can be intercourse, oral, or hand stimulation.

- **The kitchen:** She sits on the counter, he stands in front of her. Even better if you have to push dirty dishes roughly out of the way to make room.
- **The bathroom:** Standing up in the shower, in the tub, or her standing with legs apart, hands on the sink for support, as he enters from behind.
- **The powder room:** An odd choice, admittedly, but that's why it's a good choice! Pretend your parents have come for lunch and you've snuck in there while they're strolling around the garden. Add to the fantasy by leaving clothes on and simply unzipping and pulling panties to one side.
- **The laundry room:** Time it when the washing machine is on the spin cycle and it turns into a seat-size vibrator!
- **The stairs:** Doing it on the stairs is ideal if height differences stop you from using certain positions. If one stands a few steps up and the other a few steps down, heights magically even out.
- **The garage:** A sneaky way to get the thrill of doing it outside, without the complication of actually being seen by your neighbors. Just be a tad careful where you put your hands, feet—and bottoms.

Orgasm in five minutes flat

- **Use lube:** This is a must. There's no time for the vagina to lubricate naturally and sex will be painful without it.

- **Add a vibrator:** Holding a vibrator on the clitoral area is the quickest, most efficient way for a female to orgasm. If you're having oral sex, hold it against his cheek.

- **Switch stimulation:** If something doesn't feel right within a minute, try something else. Alternate between tongues, hands, intercourse, toys.

- **Do something new:** We quickly become desensitized to sexual sensations and experiences, which is why the first time for anything is often the best. New equals erotic. Add something different to your repertoire: tie each other up, wear something sexy, put on a sexy movie.

- **Do it yourself:** No one is as expert at giving you an orgasm as you are yourself. If you're finding it hard to tip over the brink, finish yourself off and suggest that your partner does the same. It doesn't mean you aren't good lovers, just that DIY gets a quicker result!

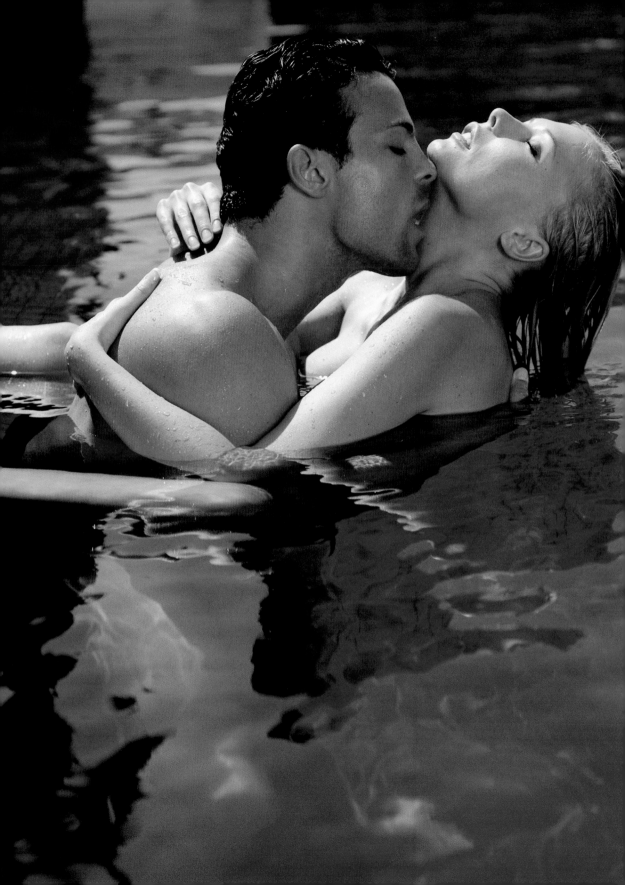

The six all-time best outdoor sex experiences

Do you score four or more?

Just as there are certain sex acts that shouldn't be missed, there are places you should have been naked in. If you can check all six boxes, you instantly win the title of Mr./Ms. Adventurous. Four shows healthy experimentation, three is usual—and anything under inexcusable. You did say you wanted great sex, didn't you? Notch a few of these up on your bedpost and you might just get it!

Nearly everyone has stumbled **half-naked into a hot tub** after a drunken dinner party. Who knew what went on **under the cover of bubbles?**

1. THE FEEL OF SUN ON NAKED FLESH

Why it feels great: Some claim the only time our bodies are truly at peace is when the sun beats down on us, because the sun's and body's biorhythms are the same. But it's not just the rays that make sex in the sun unbeatable. We're permanently worked up by a combination of sensual triggers.

People prance around in next to nothing during summer, providing a feast of flesh; a tan makes even the body-conscious feel good about being naked (as my brother says, brown fat looks better than white fat). Spreading sunscreen on each other is drop-dead sexy—continuing to rub parts that don't need it, even more so. Heat and humidity make us slow down: we're too relaxed to move, too laid-back to lift a limb, and happy to lie back and enjoy lazy, languid lovemaking... delicious!

Recreate it inside: Do it in front of the fire. Pretend you're stars of one of those cheesy 80s movies: first you'd see a bra flung on a chair, then a pair of high heels, then two half-drunk glasses of champagne. Then, finally, a couple making out on a deep sheepskin rug, fire

Vacation sex packing list:
- Condoms.
- Birth control times two (one in hand luggage, one in suitcase—try explaining "diaphragm" in Italian).
- Lube.
- Sunscreen (a sunburn stops you from touching, let alone having sex).
- Thrush cream (wet swimsuits create the perfect environment).
- Antibiotics for cystitis (nicknamed "honeymoon disease" for a reason).

sparkling prettily in the background. Yes, it *sounds* cheesy, but anyone who's tried it has to admit it *feels* extraordinary! There's a reason why those thick carpets were called "shag-pile." People spent more time lying on them than walking on them because they felt so damn comfortable. Besides, firelight is massively flattering, and being naked in front of a fire, terribly decadent. Anyone for a martini?

Swimming pools provided many women with their very first orgasm. We'd position the jet right on the clitoris and quietly climax.

2. DOING IT IN WATER OR ON THE BEACH

Why it feels great: In water, we're gloriously weightless. Everyone feels light and buoyant in mood and body (not to mention thin). The squeamish get an extra bonus: having sex in water guarantees everything is clean and fresh. Sex on the water's edge makes us feel like we're starring in *From Here to Eternity*; the smell of salt and the sea and the sound of water lapping (along with your partner) stimulate other senses. Nearly everyone's had a post liquid-dinner-party semi- (or completely) naked hot-tub experience—and even if people's toes and hands didn't accidentally float our way, the prospect was excitement enough. Swimming pools, innocent as they appear, provided many a young girl with her very first orgasm. She'd position herself so the jet of water flowed directly on her clitoris and quietly climax, appearing to be dreaming away, lost in thought.

Recreate it inside: Solo, use a hose showerhead attachment and direct the flow of water where you need it most. Try changing the water temperature (hot to cold) and strength (hard and fast to a teasing dribble) for variety. Sex in the bath or shower might not rival sex on a beach, but it comes in a sexy second place. In the shower, get her to lean back on the wall, one leg raised high, the other on the floor for balance. He supports her raised leg with his hand.

3. AT ONE WITH NATURE

Why it feels great: You're out in the middle of nowhere (a forest/desert) and suddenly you get an "I'm so happy to be alive!" rush, because it's just the two of you and Mother Nature. If you're under the shelter of a tree or in a tent, a menacing storm or copious rain only makes it even more cozy and intimate. Our libidos rise when we're outside: fresh air makes us feel energized and healthy, and the child in us associates being outdoors with freedom. As youngsters, we went outside to play "doctors and nurses," as teens to sneak our first smoke or cop a feel behind the school building. Our subconscious remembers all of this for us and taps us on the

Solve the sand-in-all-the-wrong-places problem when having sex on the beach by getting her to kneel on all fours. He kneels and then penetrates from behind.

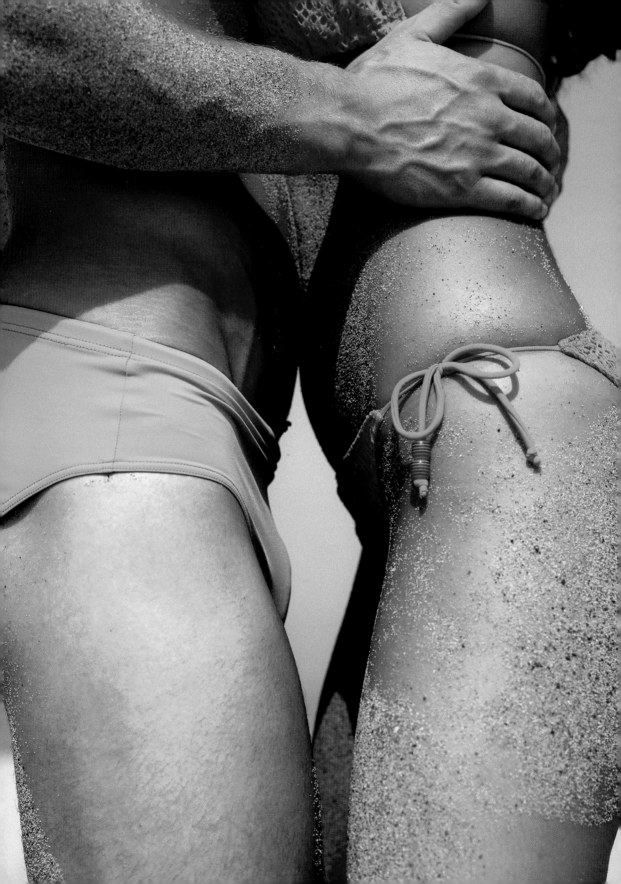

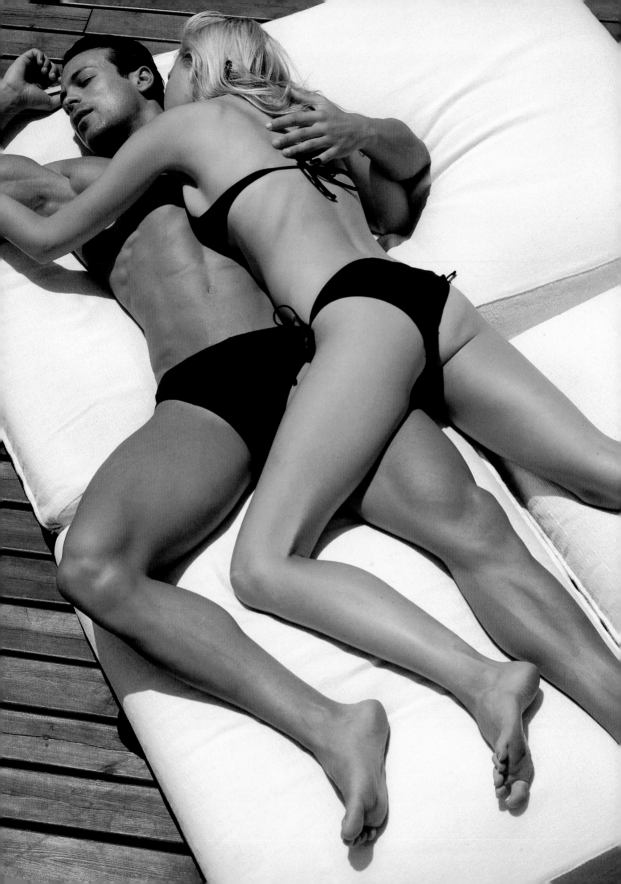

shoulder (or on another part) to remind us and to suggest we do wicked things.

Recreate it inside: Go outside when it rains, jump around like kids until you're thoroughly drenched, then go inside and have sex in the shower or the bathtub. Alternatively, pitch a tent in your yard (if you're childless, do it under cover of darkness, and if the neighbors ask about the tent, say your niece and nephew were visiting).

Posh places make us determined to make the most of where we are. We get so used to getting what we want, **the usual rules don't seem to apply.**

---

4. ON VACATION SOMEWHERE EXCLUSIVE AND EXPENSIVE

Why it feels great: Few things beat playing "LA movie producer" and sitting on a sun lounger, next to a fabulously excessive swimming pool, cocktail in hand and waiter hovering close by ready to top it off after every sip! Few of us are so rich we can loll about in luxury every day, so when we are staying somewhere glitzy, we're also in a great mood. Having already grabbed all the freebie shampoos and slugged the complimentary bubbly, you're looking for other ways to make the most of where you are. The urge to be "naughty" is strong and the elevator/hallway leading to your room/ gardens surrounding the pool morph into enormous king-size beds, begging to be romped on. You're both looking your best, making an effort to dress up for dinner, and because you're abroad and anonymous, you're more likely to do something risky. We drink more when away from home, loosening those inhibitions further, and stay up later because there's no work the next day.

Recreate it inside: If you've got some cash to spare, take yourselves out to a ritzy hotel bar or restaurant, wine and dine, then search till you find relatively private/quiet bathrooms where you can hide for a quick five minutes. If money is tight, buy one or two indulgent treats you wouldn't normally spend money on (such as gourmet chocolate, expensive wine, a rich chocolate cake, organic strawberries), climb into bed, and feed each other. Feeling spoiled and removed from the "everyday" evokes the same feelings.

5. IN A FAMOUS PLACE OR LANDMARK

Why it feels great: You're standing in front of or in a place you've been desperate to go to your whole life. Regardless of whether it's a hotel in Vegas, a balcony with a view of the Statue of Liberty, a palace, or Uncle Fred's back porch, there's enormous emotional significance attached to the

Sunshine is nature's Viagra. Levels of hormones responsible for our sex drive rise during hot weather, and sweating releases pheromones, a powerful attractant.

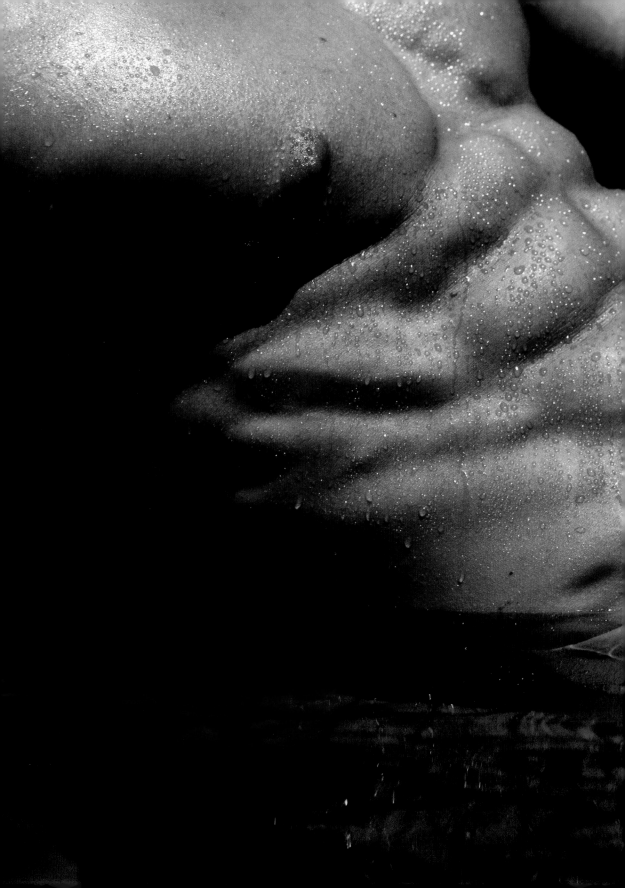

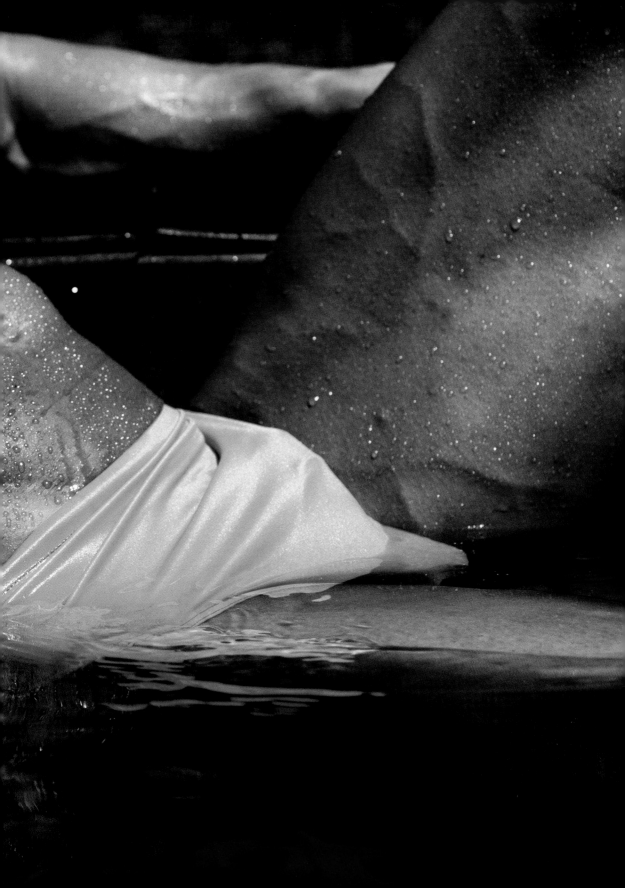

moment. Having sex in, near, or looking at a longed-for destination or landmark can turn an amazing experience into an out-of-this-world one. You're still not truly convinced you're there, so everything seems surreal and in slow motion. And even if the sex wasn't technically that great, it gets stored in the "sex experiences never to be forgotten" category because you're fulfilling a lifelong fantasy.

Try something at least three times. The first time you're concentrating on getting it right, the second, ironing out glitches, **the third... bliss!**

Recreate it inside: It sounds silly, but sometimes even watching a video or looking at photos can nudge naughty memories. Help it along by talking dirty to each other, describing what you did and how it felt at the time. Build on this to create a fantasy, adding things you wish you had done. Then plan a trip to another special place, focusing on what sort of sex you'll have there.

6. IN A CEMETERY

Why it feels great: Some of you will recoil in horror at this entry; others (the ones like me, who were obsessed with spirits, Goths, and *The Omen* as pimply youths) will completely understand. Having sex in a graveyard is the ultimate bad thing to do—which is why lots of us did it in our teens. Me included. I was going out with a minister's son (don't laugh) and one night we ended up wandering around the graveyard, drinking and smoking and having sex. Shocking now because the moral implications are clear, but at 18 I spent half my life with one finger attached to a glass hopefully placed on a Ouija board. Even if you're not a delusional teen, a cemetery makes people feel sexy because it's creepy (which makes us want to stay close) and it reminds us of our own mortality (promoting an "I might as well do it because I might be dead tomorrow" attitude). They're also often deserted, especially at night.

How to recreate it: Go to a theme park and choose a heart-stopping ride. Research shows people who go on daring dates, like skydiving, end up more attracted to the person than if they'd done the usual dinner date. Alternatively, have sex during a scary movie.

Feeling stressed and depressed? Have more sex! It seems semen contains dopamine, the "pleasure" neurotransmitter that makes us feel cuddly and snuggly. Research shows that women (in monogamous relationships) who have sex condom-free report lower levels of depression. Being touched by someone special reduces stress by reducing the level of cortisol (a hormone we produce under pressure)—so caresses also calm us.

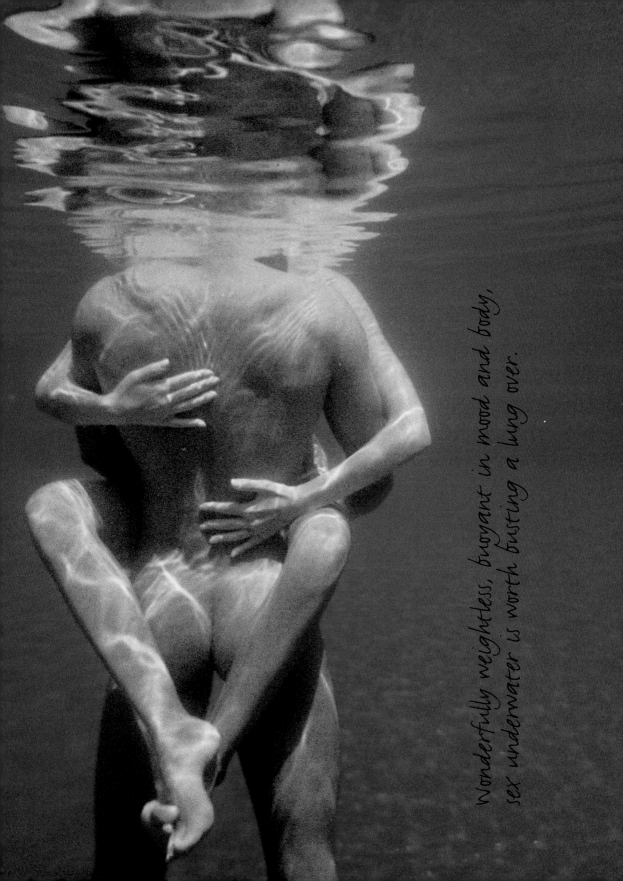

Wonderfully weightless, buoyant in mood and body, sex underwater is worth busting a lung over.

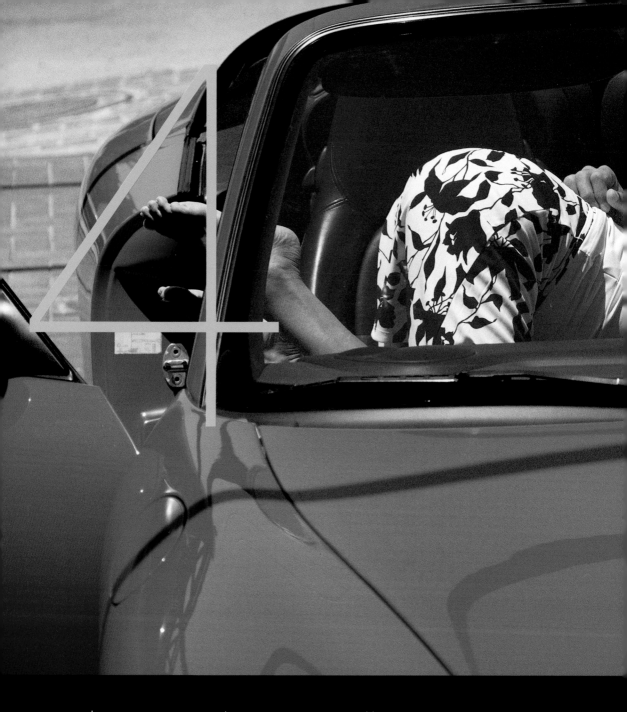

Take your sex life from dull to daring—
without ruining your relationship. Cunning ways
to up the "kink" factor and enjoy lust AND love.

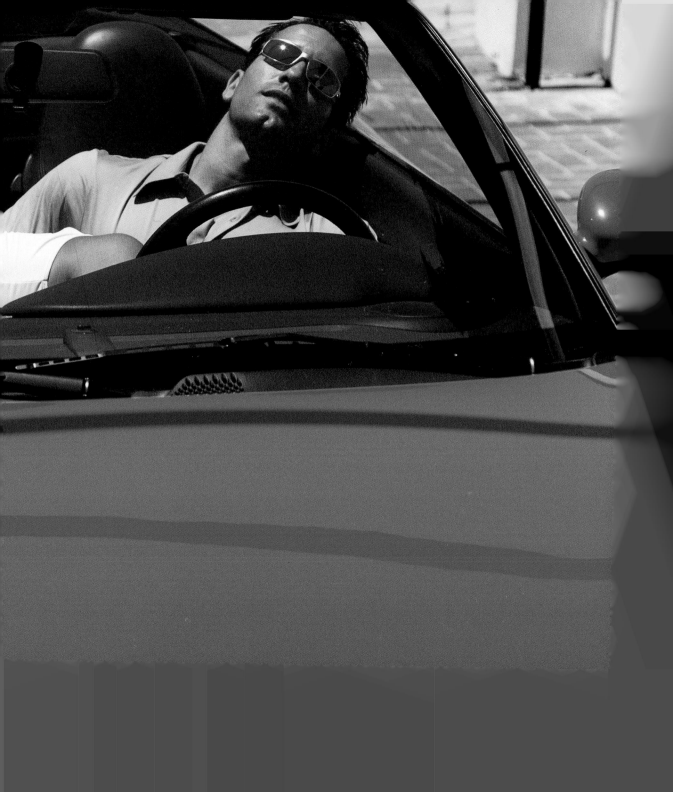

driving miss sexy

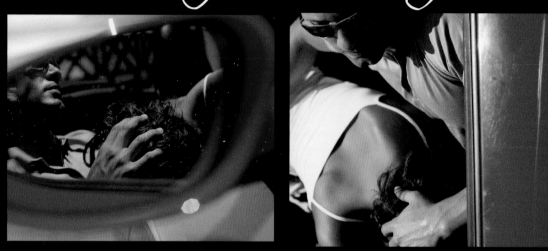

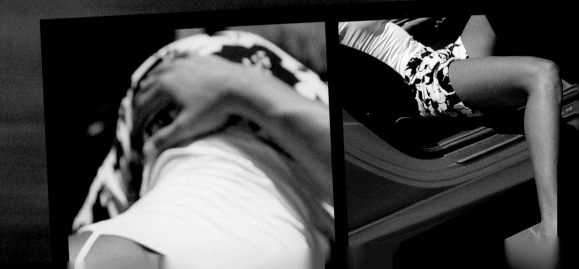

A sexy red sports car. The top off. Within seconds, his hands are inching up hers.

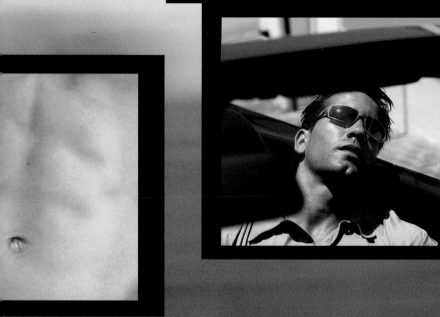
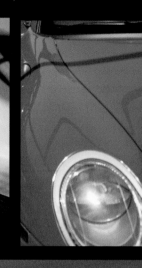
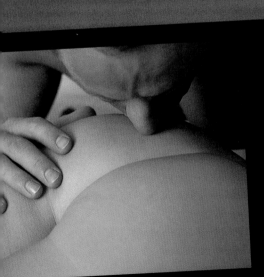
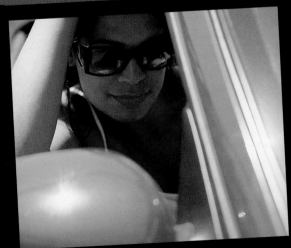
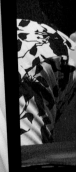

Pulled over on a deserted street, the car transforms into a bounteous boudoir.

Learn to let go and literally kick your heels up. It's totally possible to push way out of your comfort zones, without ever putting your relationship at risk.

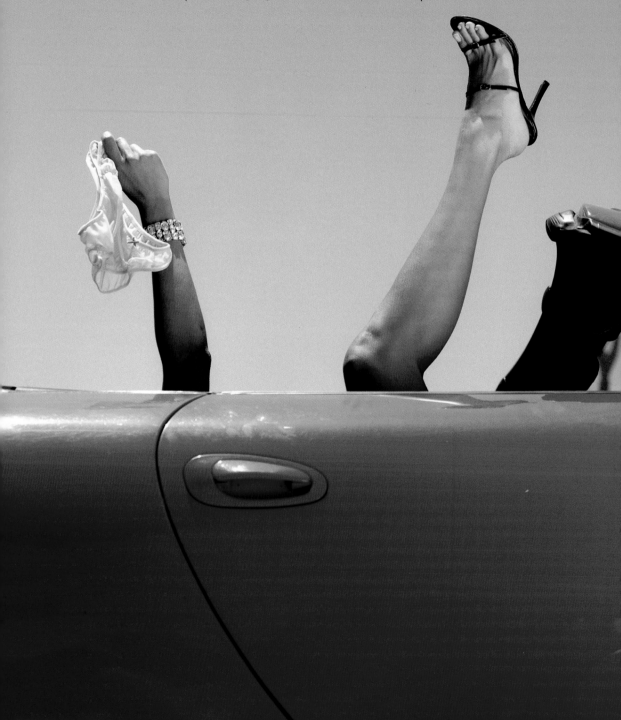

Kinky sex
Why it will save your sex and love life

One blustery winter day, I was walking down the street with an ex who'd become a good friend, about to go for Sunday lunch. It was cold, so I put my hand in my coat pocket, feeling around hopefully for a pair of gloves. "Thank God for that, I'm freezing," I said cheerily, pulling out what was in there and waving it in the air. Except it wasn't my gloves. Instead, I was waving a pair of my panties—ones I'd hastily shoved in my pocket the night before. "Oh," he said, a tad dejectedly.

It's a depressing reality that we often have **the naughtiest, raunchiest sex** with someone we don't care that much about.

"Must have been a good night last night." It was. I'd been out to dinner with my current squeeze: a guy I liked (and loved sex with), but who I had no desire to make long-term. Somewhere between the entrée and the dessert (and a few drinks), I'd brazenly removed my panties (at the table, without even attracting attention—how about that!), to allow some erotic activity underneath the tablecloth. It was edgy, dangerous, and as hot as hell. It was also something I'd never have dreamed of doing with my ex. "So how come you do that stuff with the new guy but never did with me?" my ex asked miserably a bit later. "Because I felt comfortable with you," I said. "You felt like my matching bookend." He looked confused, but sadly, I wasn't.

The best sex encounters in our lives usually aren't with people we love. This isn't just because we're worried they'll decide we're too sleazy/sordid to raise kids, it's because it's harder to have gritty sex with someone we adore. Feeling accepted, familiar, like our partner is an extension of us, makes for a fantastic relationship. But by removing all the fear and tension, sex moves from being "charged" to comfortable. Not good. As Jack Morin says in his book *The Erotic Mind*, "The messy reality is that it's harder to have good sex with someone you love. The idea that finding one's true love will automatically lead to a lifetime full of satisfying, combustible sex is a 'hearts and flowers' mentality. In truth, relationships, sex, and eroticism are infinitely more complicated."

We spend an average of two to three minutes per day having sex—and around two hours watching TV. It's clear which one we find most entertaining.

WHY BAD SEX IS GOOD SEX

Sex seems to suffer when people become closer and more compatible, possibly because we lose our sense of "otherness." We're less likely to think about our own needs and get far too caught up in satisfying theirs. However sweet and caring this is, it's not helpful when you're trying to spark fireworks rather than stoke a gently burning flame. Outrageously good sex usually has some factors we think of as "negative": guilt, rule-breaking, fear of being caught, forbidden elements, being selfish about our pleasure, doing something we know our friends would be horrified by (well, we like to think so, anyway). This type of sex usually happens in sex-for-sex's-sake relationships, one-night stands, affairs, and during risky sex with someone we really shouldn't be with. Usually. There are some couples out there who manage to balance intimacy and excitement, getting the best of both worlds. And they haven't had to compromise monogamy or pool their friends' car keys for a spot of old-fashioned swinging, to introduce these elements into a loving relationship. All they've done is upped the "kink" factor. And if you want great long-term sex, that's what you need to do.

> *Feeling depressed? Give him oral sex— and swallow. Research suggests semen acts as an antidepressant because it contains mood-improving hormones.*

BEYOND THE COMFORT ZONE

Now, before you dismiss me and my suggestion as unthinkable, hear me out. Let me first define what I mean by the word "kinky." Yes, I am talking about exploring what society brands as "taboo" sexual activities, but there's a way of doing it that doesn't involve extra bodies in the bed (see pages 132–

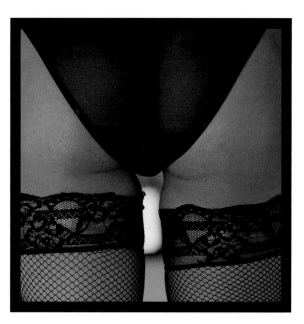

33), risking arrest, or catching something nasty. It is possible to push yourselves way out of your comfort zone without putting your relationship at risk. The aim of this book (but most particularly this chapter and the next) is to teach you how to capture the sense of "kinky," but still be sensible about it. Some things I'll suggest aren't even thought of as "out there" by most sexually adventurous people. Spanking, anal stimulation, talking dirty, blindfolds, and tie-up games—most of us have tried all or some of these things. But often not with a long-term partner—and couples who are still doing them ten years in are truly rare. My advice: bring it all back! Then introduce some other, more risqué activities. Threesomes, swinging, same-sex

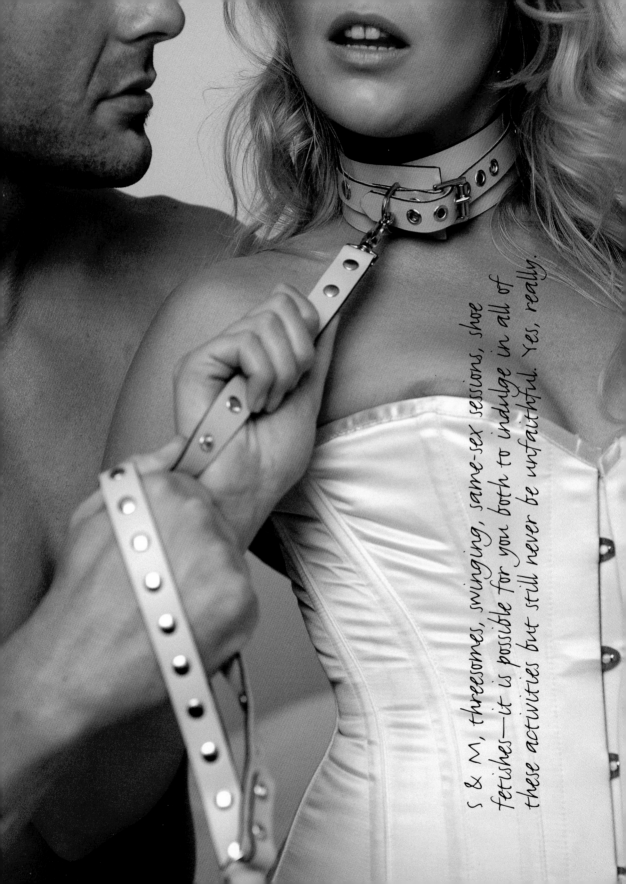

S & M, threesomes, swinging, same-sex sessions, shoe fetishes—it is possible for you both to indulge in all of these activities but still never be unfaithful. Yes, really.

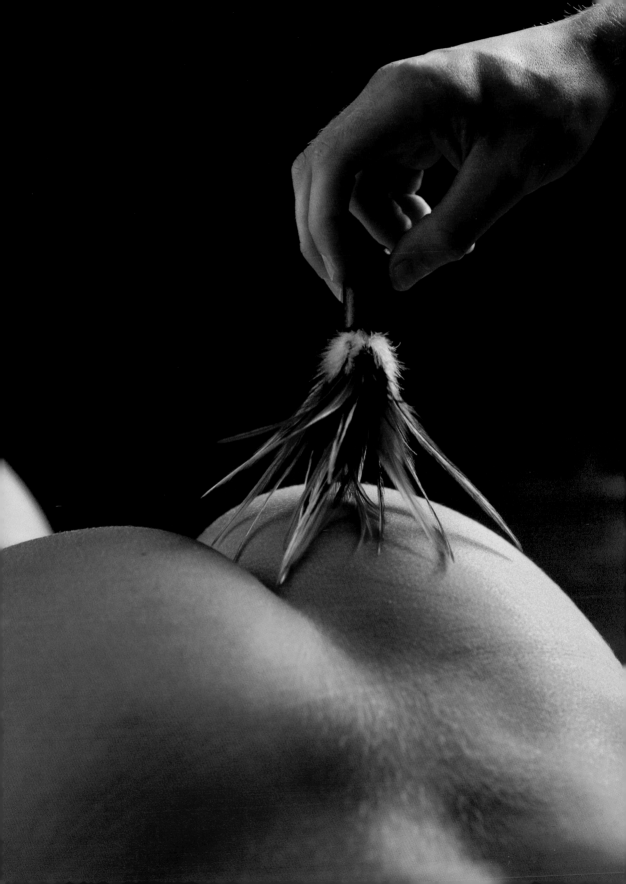

essions, fetishes—you and your partner can indulge in all of these activities but still never be unfaithful. Yes, really. It's called dipping a toe in, rather than diving in at the deep end. Doing just enough to get the heart pumping with fear and your brain throwing up thoughts like, "Should we really be doing this?" but not so much as to plague you with destructive post-event regrets.

ASK AND YOU MIGHT GET!

To put all this into practice—and in doing so transform your sex life to permanently perfect—there are two things you'll need: the right attitude and the ability to talk easily about sex with your partner. Learning how to tell your partner what you want sexually is one of the most challenging and rewarding skills you can develop. You need to ditch the notion, however romantic, that they'll intuitively know how to please you because they love you. Or that you'll hurt their feelings by wanting more than they're providing. Most men pray for the suggestion of any form of sexual variety and often feel condemned for daring to want it. They're constantly being told that to satisfy their partners, they have to make love like a woman. But however many rose petals he scatters across the bed, it's still only going to produce "Oh, sweetheart!" feelings of love, not the jangly, frenzied, fervid stirrings of passion I'm talking about here. Women are slightly less open to risky activities—but more because we've been brainwashed to think they are "unladylike" than out of lack of desire to try them. Put us in a loving, open, trusting relationship where we know we're not going to be judged, and we can be just as down-and-dirty as the boys.

For a moment, try forgetting what your mother/the church/your bossy big sister and brother/your boring ex-partner/preachy, puritanical papers have told you. Wipe the slate clean and imagine a world where anything (that doesn't cause you or your partner emotional or unwanted physical pain) goes. Read, discuss, and then put some of the suggestions in this chapter into practice, see what results you get, then move on to the next one. Try the things that instantly appeal first, then give the other stuff a shot—just for the hell of it. Make sure you play fair (see pages 24–25), accept that you'll occasionally have misunderstandings and probably arguments as you both adjust to the new, more honest versions of yourselves, don't expect to enjoy everything you try, and you might be *very* happy with what happens.

Above all, remember to balance all those lusty sessions with lots of love and emotional intimacy. They really don't have to be mutually exclusive!

Forty percent of people who admit to being embarrassed to talk sex with their partner are dissatisfied with their sex life.

In a major magazine survey of 100,000 married women, the strongest indicator of sexual and marital satisfaction was the wives' ability to express sexual feelings to their husbands. The more they talked, the better they rated their sex lives, their marriages, and their overall happiness.

Bottoms up!
A bit of slap-and-tickle could be just what you need

I never really "got" the spanking thing, until I visited a specialty shop during the filming of one of my TV shows. The couple we were working with were eager to try spanking, so I dutifully but dubiously trotted along with the female partner to investigate...

Once inside, we were like women with a bad case of PMS, let loose in Willy Wonka's chocolate factory. Pink sparkly riding crops, soft-as-silk whips, which whooshed through the air but tickled rather than hurt, predatory paddles—wide-eyed, we loved them all, transforming ourselves into circus animal tamers and spanking the bottoms of all the crew (most particularly the gorgeous sound guy, who could barely sit down at dinner!). "Spank me!", I was soon shouting, while the owner of the shop smiled smugly behind the counter, having heard my initial claims of "it does nothing for me." Not only was it damn good fun, the feeling of power produced an unexpected, arousing adrenaline rush.

Theories on why a slap on the bottom feels sexy abound. Some say it's the result of humiliating childhood spanking sessions. When something bad happens to us as a child, we naturally try to turn it into something positive. The shame of being bent over a (sexy) teacher's knee in front of the class is turned into an erotic episode so the child can cope. Later on, a playful slap from a lover subconsciously reignites that feeling. Spanking is also a turn-on because "hurting" each other is unacceptable—this makes it forbidden (and an instant aphrodisiac). Then there's the link between pleasure and pain—a well-placed, well-timed slap on the bottom feels good, as I found out! Pain is one of the strongest sensations you can feel—and it doesn't diminish once you're accustomed to it. Light and consistent stroking is screened out by our subconscious; pain stays in our awareness. As with any new sexual activity, there are ways to try it out sensibly and safely. Read on...

THE STROKE-BY-STROKE GUIDE
- **Don't even think** about starting the session until they're fully aroused. The more erotically aroused they are, the more likely they are to be receptive to erotic pain. Stop spanking the minute their arousal level falls.
- **Run your fingers lightly over their buttocks**, tickling them. Then place one hand on a buttock cheek, the other on the genitals. Start with the cheek closest to you.
- **Cup your hand** slightly, keeping your fingers together and spank in a slightly upward motion. This feels better than a downward stroke. Keep your wrist flexible to begin with—experiment by holding it rigid a little later on.

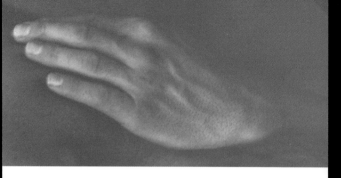

- **Your first spank** should be more like a caress than a slap. After you've dispensed it, massage the area for a few seconds and fondle the genitals.
- **Then try another spank,** timing them to arrive no more than three to five seconds apart. Cover both cheeks, aiming for the lower (fleshier) part of the cheeks, and start to increase the force. Vary the weight, frequency, and placement of the slaps.
- **Later, try dispensing a spank,** then holding your hand still on the skin for a second or so. Rub, stroke, or lick the area for a further second, before giving another spank.
- **Alternate the spank of your hand** with a different texture—a fur mitt, the back of a hairbrush. Or contrast the slap of spanking with light, feathery strokes or kisses.
- **A vibrator** held between her legs (by clamping her thighs shut) doubles the stimulation.
- **Use an ice cube** to cool down the skin after a spank. Then lick or rub the area to provide the contrast of hot and cold.

SPANK SENSIBLY

Have keywords or signals to show whether the person is happy with the level of pain. A nod or "yes" could mean they're enjoying it but don't want it any harder; "more" or "now" means up the intensity level. To judge how hard to hit, get your partner to rate each slap on a scale of 1–10. One is very light, 10 is hard. Start gently, then build up, with them calling out the number that corresponds with the stroke. Let them decide on the number they're most comfortable with. If "4" suits them but they then want more or less, they call out "3" (for lighter) or "5" (for stronger).

How to suggest it

Some people think it's degrading to spank their partner. Which it definitely is, if you don't ask for it and they suddenly start slapping you! But wanting them to spank you is quite another thing. Because spanking involves pain, asking someone to spank you is scary! So what do you do, when you know what you want but don't know how to get it? Here's a few tricks:

- Test the waters by gauging their reactions to mild pain. When they're next aroused, pinch their nipples slightly, then harder and watch how they react. Do they shout "Ouch!" and glare at you? This is a red light. If, however, they gasp but their breathing stays deep and slow, they could be open to it. A little involuntary moan is a flashing green light! Bear in mind some people like some types of pain but not others—they might hate their nipples bitten but love a well-delivered slap on the bottom. If the nipple-pinching doesn't work, next time playfully slap them on the bottom, seeing what effect that has.

- If you're fairly confident they won't pack their bags at the suggestion, slip them a sexy note, saying what you're going to do later (they've been naughty and you're going to punish them) or buy a soft whip as a present. Worried they'll think you're a pervy deviant? Find a sexy spanking scene in an erotic book, then read it to your partner. If they look at you like you just read out something akin to an orgy with their grandparents, simply shrug and say, "Well, I thought it was sort of sexy."

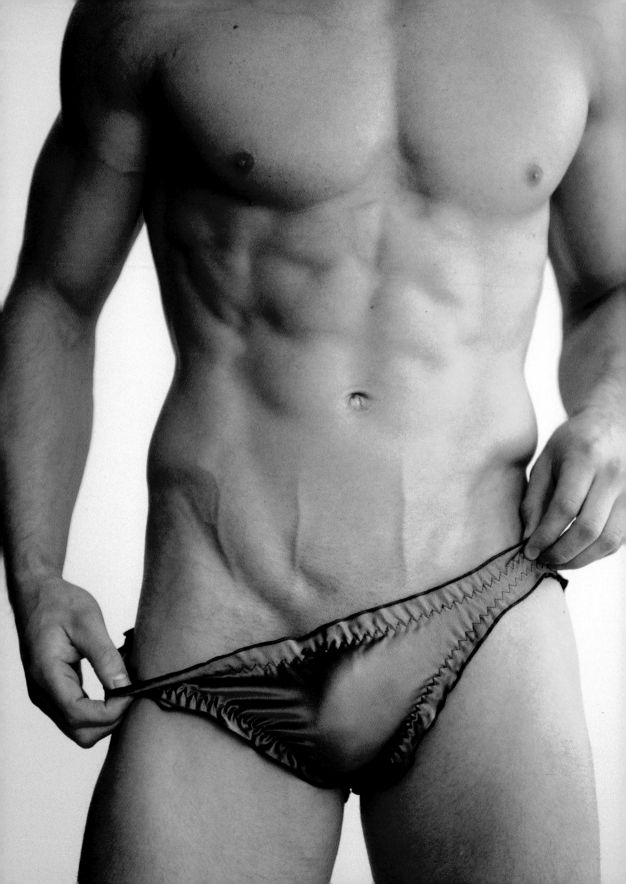

Taboo territory
Dipping a toe in...

Having (at least semi- ?) convinced you of the benefits of breaking out of a predictable pattern of lovemaking, it's time to make some suggestions. Despite the rather scary subheadings (Cross-dressing? Yikes!), there's really nothing too demanding here. So push aside any negative gut reactions, snuggle up on the couch with a stiff drink, and see if anything else follows suit.

When it comes to **wanting sex,** men tend to be on a five-day cycle, while women edge toward ten. But it's also true that **the more varied the sex,** the more both of **you will want it.**

BONDAGE AND TIE-UP GAMES

B & D (bondage and domination) is a tamer version of S & M (sadomasochism)—less leather masks and studded collars, more high heels, sexy lingerie, and pairs of old stockings. Lots of us have been tied to the odd four-poster bed in our time—and most like it. Being tied up appeals because it increases the suspense of sexual pleasure: you can't control when someone touches, teases, licks, or penetrates you, and you are "forced" to give in (handily removing any sexual guilt). If you're in the power position, you get the enormous kick of having someone completely at your sexual mercy—it's spectacularly politically incorrect, which is why we love it so much!

Some people don't stop at tying up—they assume even more power by gagging their partners as well, but this takes domination through to another level. It's one thing having your arms tied behind your head, quite another not being able to say, "Hey, I'm bored with this now. Untie me!"

If you're the type to lie back and take it, rather than take command, try something new. Touch your partner before they touch you. Make your strokes firmer and authoritative. Say "Go down on me" rather than pushing their head southward. Choose positions where you're in control, and instead of lying back during oral sex, sit on his face or get her to kneel in front of you. Direct your partner on how to pleasure you.

If you're adventurous, try this:

- She's on her hands and knees; he ties her feet and hands and then enters her from behind. As she "struggles," she pushes back against him, increasing the pleasure.
- She ties him up and sits astride him, facing away. Firmly grasping the root of his penis with one hand, she uses the other to stroke upward rapidly. Stopping for one second every three, she keeps going until he's about to climax, then climbs on top to finish him off.

Having someone **completely at your sexual mercy** is spectacularly **politically incorrect**, which is **why we love it** so much!

Wimp's way out:

- Test the waters: if someone's not sure how they'll feel being tied up, hold their wrists together above their head with your hands during sex or instruct them to keep their hands behind their backs or they'll get "in trouble."
- Make it plain it's a fun tie-up session, rather than serious S & M. If they're really nervous, tie them up with toilet paper, which gives the feeling of being held hostage without any threat (at all). Using everyday objects—like socks, scarves, or old stockings—makes it seem less threatening than serious-looking handcuffs or hard rope.

PLAYING SAFELY

- Don't use knots that tighten if the tied-up person struggles, and make sure it feels comfortable for them by slipping one finger between the bond and their wrist or ankle before tightening knots.
- Keep a pair of scissors or the key to handcuffs handy in case they (or you) have a sudden "Get me out!" panic.
- Never keep someone tied up for more than half an hour—especially if they smoke or drink heavily. (It's not good for poor circulation.)
- It should be common sense never to suspend anyone by their wrists, ankles, or neck (that's called autoerotic asphyxiation—something I DON'T recommend!).
- If you're using a gag, make sure the person can breathe and make a noise.
- Never—no matter how funny you think it would be—leave someone tied up alone in a room. This isn't the time to run out for a gallon of milk.

True virtual sex isn't far away. We'll soon climb into sex suits, fitted with stimulators in erogenous zones, and watch movies, able to experience what we're seeing.

What to do when you've got them trussed up? Absolutely anything and everything—touch, lick, kiss, and penetrate, with a heavy emphasis on tease.

CROSS-DRESSING

Ever noticed how men are always more enthusiastic about costume parties where the sexes swap clothes? She grumbles and makes half-hearted attempts with a tie and a stick-on mustache; he rifles through her closet and chooses the biggest, dangliest earrings he can find, seconds after the invitation arrives. There's a good reason why—and it doesn't mean he's gay. Women can dress as men any time they like (bar the mustache), but it's not acceptable for men to wear women's clothes. Slinky skirts, butt-skimming minis, high heels, silky panties, push-up bras, stockings, and garter belts are all banned from his bod. Given an excuse to try it, is it any wonder even the butchest boys are up for it? And it's not just women's clothes they steal. Swishing their hair, touching up their makeup, they adopt feminine mannerisms as well. They're curious (and often jealous) of women's sexual power, and this offers a chance to see how it feels. But it's one thing having a giggle at a costume party, quite another to open your lingerie drawer and find your Victoria's Secrets stretched beyond recognition.

> *seventy five percent of cross-dressers are heterosexual. It's about transformation: satisfying a curiosity about what it would feel like to be the opposite sex.*

It's one thing having a giggle at a costume party, quite another to open your lingerie drawer to find your **Victoria's Secrets stretched beyond recognition.**

Cross-dressing (men wanting to wear women's clothes—usually underwear—for sexual pleasure) has been around forever, but came to the fore a few years ago when some prominent "real men" confessed to doing it. Seventy five percent of cross-dressers are heterosexual. In fact, it is only considered a problem if it becomes an entrenched fetish (when sex or arousal is impossible without it) or if their partner dislikes it so much that it's ruining the relationship. To be honest, I don't know any women who want their partner to be a cross-dresser. It makes us feel uneasy (not to mention protective of our pantyhose). However, a couple I know were messing around and she made him put on her silk panties. She manipulated the silk around his penis to give an exquisite hand-job. Because he wasn't used to the feel of silk (being resigned to boring old cotton boxer shorts), he rated it as one of the sexiest sessions ever. Try it! If you both like it, get him to wear a pair of your girliest panties next time you go out. Even a trip to the mall becomes edged with excitement. You both share a wicked secret (though he should avoid low-slung Levi's if you want to keep it that way), and the unusual feel of slippery fabric against his private parts is a constant reminder of what's in store later.

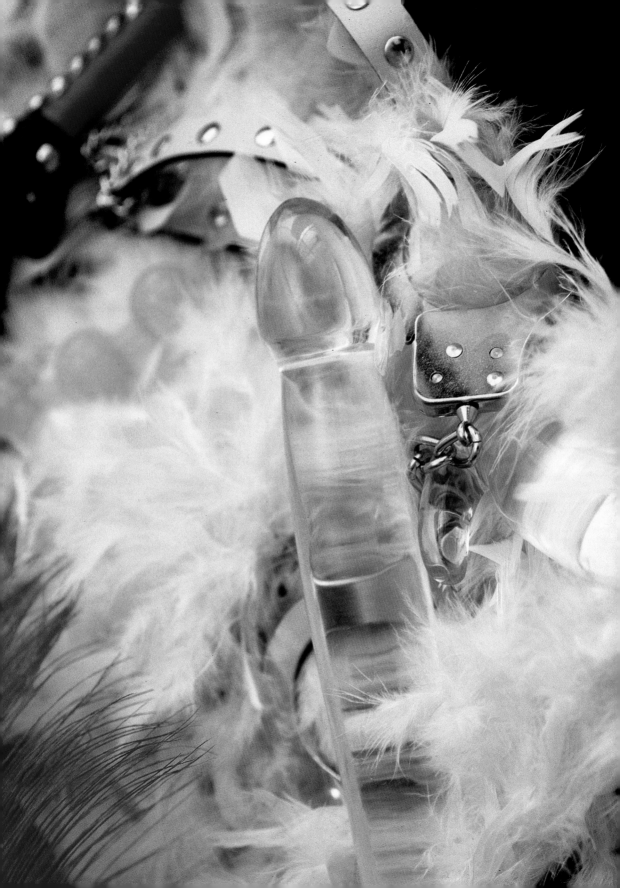

Kinky confessional
Some straight answers

My boyfriend told me it would really turn him on if I wet my panties in front of him. He says loads of people do it.

Urophilia—a sexual interest in urine—isn't common sexual behavior (so your boyfriend's pulling your leg with his every-second-guy-on-the-bus-wants-it claim). On the other hand, it's not rare. Why would he enjoy it? Sexologists think it could result if urine and arousal get linked when the person is very young, at the time they're forming their "sexual blueprint." When we first experience sexual feelings, often the events surrounding it tend to influence how we'll make love in the future. For instance, your boyfriend could have been scolded by his mom for wetting his pants when he was a child and been locked in his bedroom. Bored, he started messing around and ending up masturbating for the first time—and that's how the two got linked together. If it's kept as an occasional thing and you both enjoy it, I don't see a problem (though your cleaning lady might). What could be an issue is if he wants to do it all the time. You may then feel he's more interested in the peeing than in you.

I'm being hassled by my boyfriend to shave off my pubic hair. Should I do it, and if so how?!

How or if you wax, shave, or trim is highly personal. I slept with a guy who shaved everything, including his testicles. This struck me as odd because it didn't go with his personality: he was kind of shy and (claimed) he wasn't that sexually confident. Since then, I've discovered it's now de rigueur in that age group (18–25). Letting a person shave you is an incredibly sexy exercise (even if it does itch like crazy afterward). It involves trust and it exposes the genitals. Penises and vaginas look "naked" and vulnerable without hair (that reddish blush isn't just from sexual arousal, they're embarrassed!). Some people think removing all hair from the female genitalia has sinister connotations, because it mimics a young girl. In 99.9 percent of cases, that's not the case. Hair in your mouth is a pain, being able to see clearly what you're doing is a bonus. But be careful, whatever hair removal method you use. I was trimming my pubic hair with sharp scissors once, one

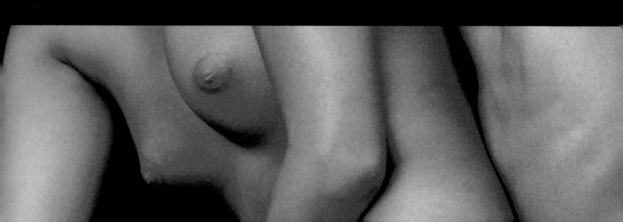

leg up on the toilet seat, my phone tucked under my chin as I talked to my boyfriend. Multi-tasking is admirable, but sometimes not wise. Next thing I know, a huge lump of labia dropped in my hand. Like, owww! Another friend was trimming his testicles while watching the football when his team scored. He claims he went through two rolls of toilet paper trying to mop up the mess. Not sexy.

What exactly is deep-throating, and is it something every woman can learn?

Most of the sensation of the penis is in the head and the frenulum (the little stringy bit) so making six inches disappear, like a circus sword-swallower, is unnecessary. All it really does is dispense a pleasant psychological kick by allowing him to indulge his porn-star fantasy. But if you're feeling particularly generous, try this technique. To deep throat, you have to widen the natural ninety-degree angle of your throat by choosing specific positions. If you lie on your back, your head hanging off the edge of the bed, with him either standing or kneeling by the side of the bed, you can use your hands against his thighs to control the depth. It's worth giving it a shot for the pure novelty factor, but if it results in unpleasant gagging rather than a mind-blowing orgasm, don't blame me!

When people talk about cybersex, do they simply mean strangers masturbating in a chatroom?

The online sex industry generates one billion US dollars a year—for a reason. You can access websites, information, and pictures on virtually anything your wicked little mind can conjure up, all in the privacy of your own home. But cybersex isn't just about two strangers pounding away at their keyboard (simultaneously pounding other things). There's a lot couples can do online sexually. Grab a drink, log on, and have some fun! As well as trawling the net for whatever porn takes your fancy, you can use it to solve any sex problems (there are tons of advice sites) or look for ideas of new things to try. One or both of you can visit a naughty chatroom, flirting with each other or other people. It's a safe, saucy way for secure couples to let loose those infidelity urges that affect us all. (Emphasis on the word "secure": some people get nervous watching their partner in full seduction mode.) You can be as explicit as you like and assume any persona: he gets to be a girl and you a guy. Also check out "strip sites," where you pay to spy on people in their bedrooms, getting up to all sorts of things.

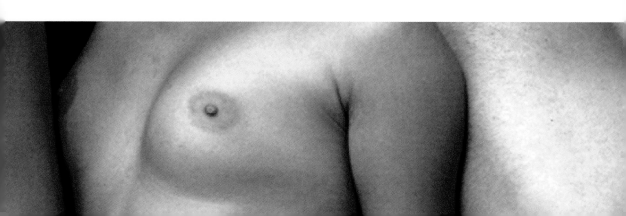

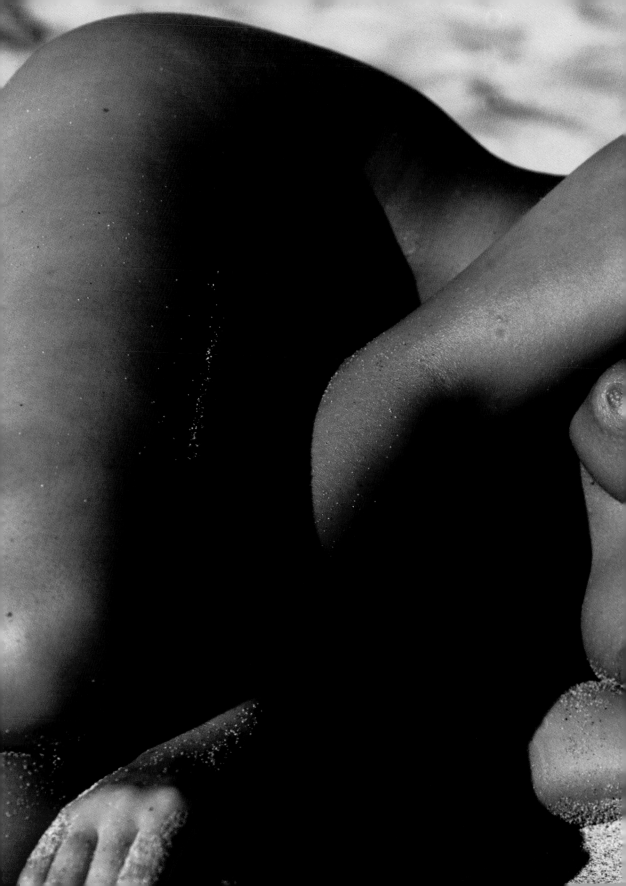

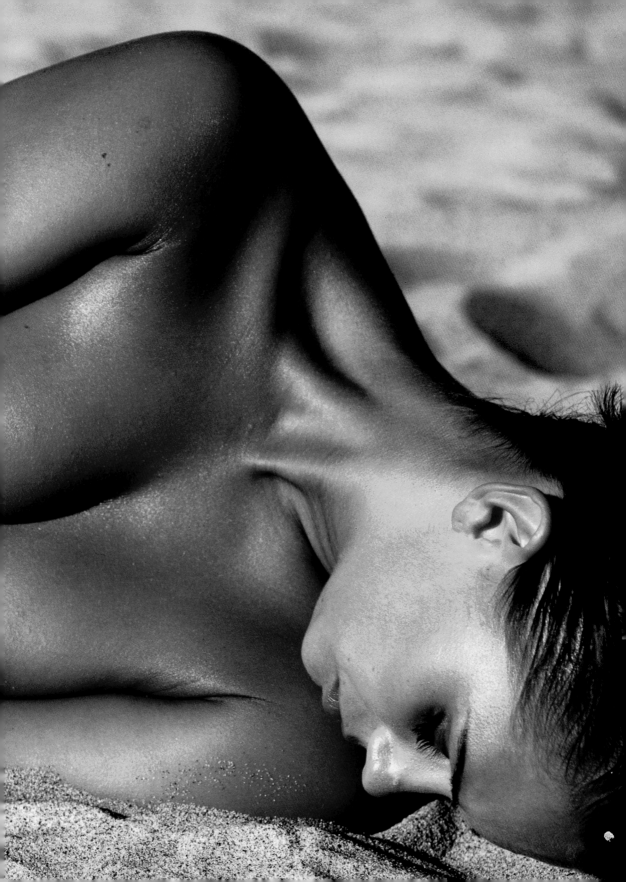

Going in the back door
Safe, sensible anal sex

Despite being wildly popular with the Greeks in the good old orgy days, anal sex was something men wanted and women avoided until recently. Now both sexes are happily exploring "backdoor" sex.

Kinsey reported in 1990 that 11 percent of married men had tried anal sex or had it regularly. More recent research found that 30–40 percent of heterosexual couples had tried it, with up to half doing it regularly. (Interestingly, while 2.5 million straight US couples are said to practice anal sex, only about 50 percent of gay men do the same.) There's usually no "wrong" way to have sex, but when it comes to anal sex, you need to be informed for it to be as painless as possible. Here are some tips...

How do I talk her into trying it?

Plenty of women enjoy anal sex—if, and it's a big if—it's done properly. What puts most of us off is having had the old, "Ooops, I got the wrong hole" trick pulled on us. "Accidentally" and eagerly thrusting into an unlubricated, unprepared anus hurts like hell. And it's put plenty of women off for life. The second most likely thing to put us off is your asking for it over and over again, which (like the threesome request) only makes us more determined not to do it. A playful suggestion that you'd like to try it—along with a "you don't have to if you don't want to, but I'd at least like to try stimulating you with my finger"—will get you further. I'd also suggest backing up your suggestion with some good articles to allay her fears. Gently remind her just because something is seen as culturally "taboo," doesn't mean it is. Not so long ago, it was "unnatural" for women to work and only "whores" gave oral sex. Things constantly move from "bizarre" to mainstream once society's attitudes relax or change. Anal sex is one of them.

Will she enjoy it?

Approached properly, anal sex can be intensely pleasurable for her. The rectum shares a wall with the vagina and penetrating it gives a pleasant feeling of fullness in both the vagina and anus. It's also seen as taboo (always a turn-on). The naughtiness of a finger inside her anus, another inside the vagina, and an expert tongue rates up there as one of life's greatest pleasures. Can she orgasm purely through anal? Most sex experts say no. Anal sex could, however, tip her over into orgasm if she's hovering on the brink (even better, if you're stimulating her clitoris while inside her).

Will it hurt?

Not if done properly. The process of anal sex needs to be slow because the anal sphincter muscles are used to pushing things out, not taking anything in. You must use lubrication—silicone-based, not water—and relax the muscles by massaging with your fingers first. Anal sex nearly always feels uncomfortable initially, but once you relax into it the pain should subside. If, however, the pain is

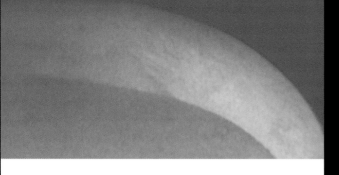

sharp, shooting, or if it feels like something is tearing, you're not doing it right. Slow down, add more lube, and don't thrust too hard.

But that's where poop comes from!

The rectum is a passageway, not a storage place. The anal canal is less than an inch long, the rectum is between five and nine inches long, and this in turn leads to the colon—which is where the feces accumulate. But the more recently you've gone to the bathroom, the less likely you are to get an unpleasant surprise. Invest in some soap-free solutions (any that are marketed for feminine use) and insert a soapy finger during your shower. Have unscented baby wipes on hand during any anal play, put down some dark-colored towels, and if you're particularly squeamish (or worried about infection), use latex gloves for finger insertion or condoms for intercourse.

Will I catch anything?

Anal play can spread HIV and other sexually transmitted infections. It's also possible to get pregnant from anal sex if the semen slides into the vagina. Protect yourselves by getting tested for STDs, and by using condoms, a latex glove for finger insertion, and a cut-up condom or plastic wrap for rimming (see page 182). Don't put anything that has been in the anus into the vagina without thoroughly washing it first.

What positions are best?

Try missionary (she's on her back, knees pulled to her chest, with her feet on his shoulders); rear entry (she's lying on her stomach, using pillows to raise her bottom); her on top (she straddles him and sits on his penis). The classic porn pose is for her to stand and bend over.

Tips for the first-timer

If you're the person penetrating:

- Never go straight into penile penetration without having tried other stuff first (fingers, dildos, vibrators).
- Apply LOTS of lube to both your penis and her bottom, then rub the penis head against her opening.
- Wait for the anus to relax and open and let her back onto your penis, rather than do the penetrating yourself.
- Hold your penis at the base and wait until the head (only) penetrates. Pause until she says it's OK to go further and insert a little at a time, very slowly.
- Once it's all in, pause again, then do slow, gentle thrusts. Angle yourself so you're aiming for her belly button.
- Stop regularly to apply more lubrication and exit as slowly as you entered—go too fast, and the muscles will tense and spasm.

If you're on the receiving end:

- The more aroused you are, the less it will hurt (though having an orgasm first can also relax you).
- Hold your bottom open and bear down (as though you're trying to go to the toilet)—this opens your anus.
- Breathe deeply, then back up to allow him to penetrate a little. If you start to panic, try contracting your anal muscles voluntarily to give you a sense of control.
- Give him constant feedback. It can take a few sessions before you can accept him fully, so don't feel rushed or pressured.

Toy story
It's playtime...

Having just launched my own sex toy range, I can safely boast that I've pretty much tried them all. Quite apart from testing the limits of my long-suffering cleaner, who faithfully dusted the 16 "rabbits" lined up neatly on the desk ready for future testing, it was interesting to see how my then-boyfriend reacted to this research.

"I'm exhausted," I complained. "I've just had three orgasms in a row, and I've got another eight vibrators to test." Silence at the other end, rather than sympathy. "Two more than you usually have with me," he said grumpily, threatening to picket my apartment building with a "Save the Males" sign. Oddly, sex toy shopping is one area where women are far more adventurous than men. Yes, it is shopping (which explains a lot), but it's also because men see things like vibrators as "replacements" rather than additions to a sex life. They're not—and there are good reasons why men should encourage their partners to own one (see page 26). Sex toys are as the name suggests—things to play with for a bit of fun! And have fun you will!

Walking into a sex shop can be bewildering, so I've compiled a list of the items you're likely to be drawn to. You can use this to shop online if you're shy (and yes, they will arrive in brown packaging, not a bag that screams "10-INCH THROBBING DILDO!"). But I'd highly recommend you visit a reputable sex shop together so that you can pick the products up, feel, and test them. It's also a naughty, sexy thing to do! Choose your shop depending on your mood—a suitably sleazy one if you're feeling down and dirty, a "posh" shop (and there are plenty if you search online), or even "women's only" if he wants to lurk around the corner. If you're paranoid you'll run into his sister, choose one in an area she's unlikely to visit. If you get caught and they look aghast, launch straight into a funny story of what happened in there. That makes them look like a prude and you wonderfully liberated! Research suggests around 10 percent of adults use sex toys regularly, I'd put that much higher. Around 60 percent of my girlfriends own a vibrator (and they're seriously not weird, honest!).

Dominate me...
BLINDFOLDS—Something safe to pounce on—you know what it is and what to do with it! You can make a blindfold out of anything, but fancy ones are good for role-play and dress-up.
WHIPS, RIDING CROPS, AND PADDLES—Each designed to produce different types of pain: whips are softest, riding crops medium, and paddles hurt.

LET'S GO SHOPPING!

Vibrators—Every woman's best friend, vibrators come in all shapes and sizes, from a buzzing lipstick to a throbbing 10-inch fleshlike (terrifying) thing. Narrow the selection by deciding what you want from yours: if it's for masturbation and you're into penetration with clitoral stimulation, go for a "rabbit" (a penis-shaped vibrator with a clitoral attachment). "Wand" vibrators—small cylindrical vibrators that you hold against the clitoris—are ideal for use during intercourse. For more powerful clitoral vibration, opt for one that looks like a back massager—large with a big rounded head (like the Hitachi Magic Wand). Choose from small, hard plastic ones (better vibration) or jellylike rubber or silicone varieties (weaker vibration but feel nicer). Make sure you get one with variable speed. Test how quiet it is and check if it's waterproof if you want to use it in the tub or shower. "Butterfly" vibrators are attached via elastic leg straps and provide clitoral stimulation during intercourse, but a wand vibrator held in place works just as well. (For more info on vibrator techniques, see page 26.)

Dildos—These are imitation penises of varying sizes. Unlike vibrators, they don't vibrate. Usually made of rubber, they're sometimes S-shaped for G-spot stimulation. If you like the feeling of fullness, they're good to insert during oral sex. You'll also see strap-on versions called "harnesses," which are attached via thigh and bottom straps and transform her into a him instantly—the ultimate gender-bender! Some women feel powerful popping on a phallus. I tried one on once and felt more like a carpenter with a tool belt on—and ruined the mood completely by walking around being cocky (literally), imagining what it would be like to be a man.

Anal toys—Anal vibrators have a flared base (so what goes up doesn't disappear). Butt plugs are soft, jellylike, and stay in better, but don't vibrate. Anal beads are plastic balls attached to a thin nylon cord. The idea is to insert them, then pull them out (not too fast) right before or during orgasm.

Vibrating penis rings—Traditional penis rings slip on to a flaccid or semi-erect penis. They trap blood in the penis, helping him to maintain a stronger erection for longer, and make the penis look and feel bigger. The vibrating versions are a great invention—they're inexpensive as well. These are penis rings—usually rubber—with little vibrators attached for clitoral stimulation. In order for them to work effectively, though, he uses a grinding, circular thrusting motion during intercourse and rides high to keep the little vibrator in contact with the clitoris as much as possible.

S & M GEAR—Those menacing-looking studded collars, leather outfits, and masks are sometimes enough to send you scuttling out the door. Intrigued rather than intimidated? See page 127, for a feature on the topic.
NIPPLE CLAMPS—These clip onto your nipples to create the sensation of pinching (i.e., pain). S & M devotees adore them. The rest of us look at them, think "Ouch!" and then move back to the warm, fuzzy vibrator section.

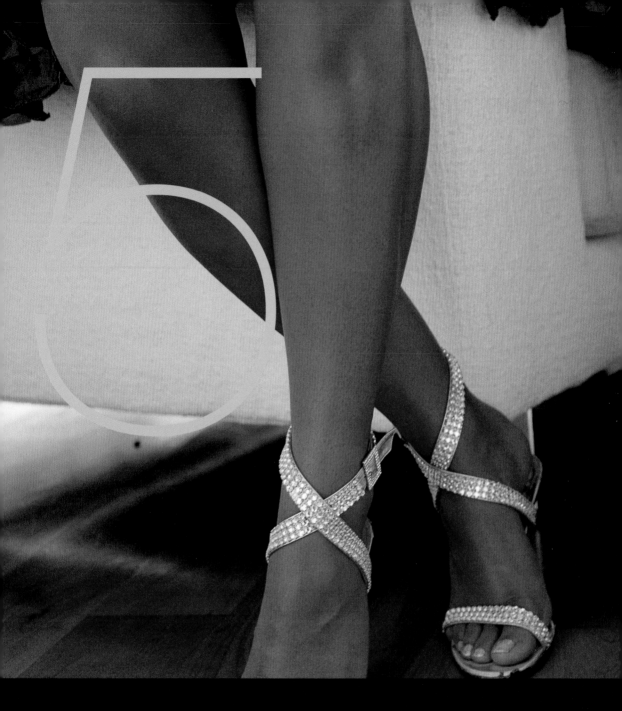

5

Rev things up a gear (or three) by indulging in all those super-seedy sex scenarios you'd secretly lo to try. Yes, you can do it and stay faithful too!

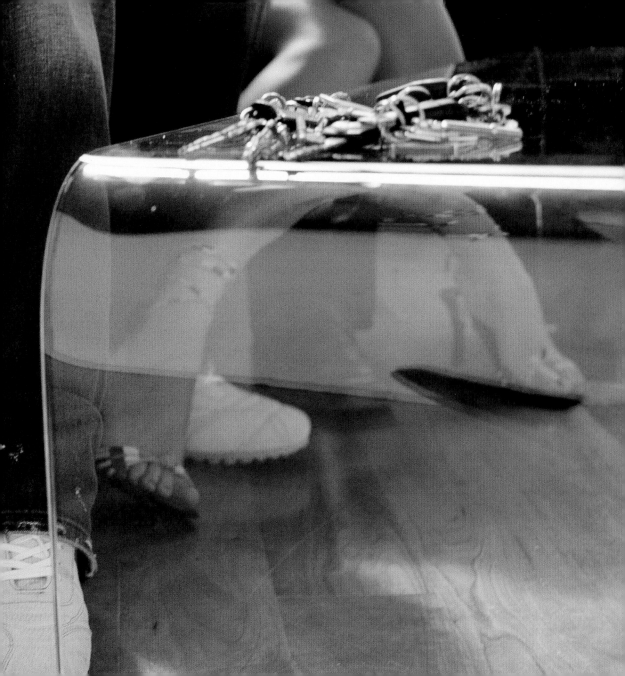

hedonist's heaven

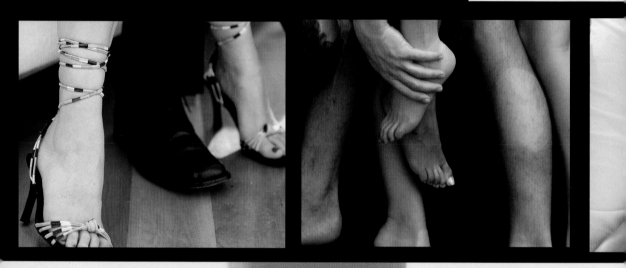

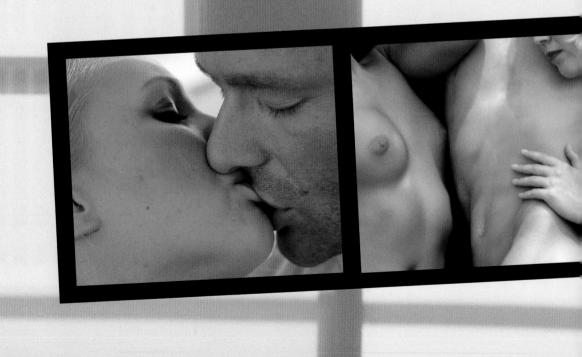

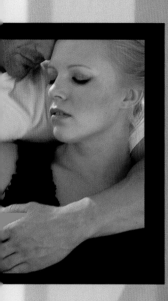

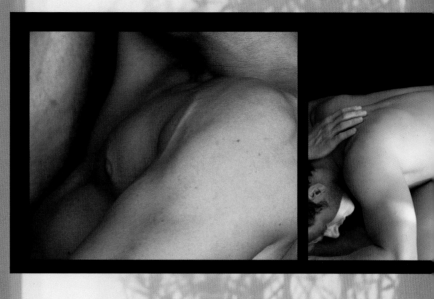

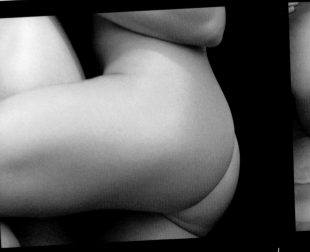

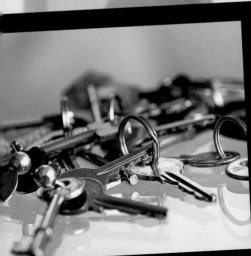

Bodies stroking, sucking, indulging in a sensual, sensory feast. (Shame it's not like that in real life!)

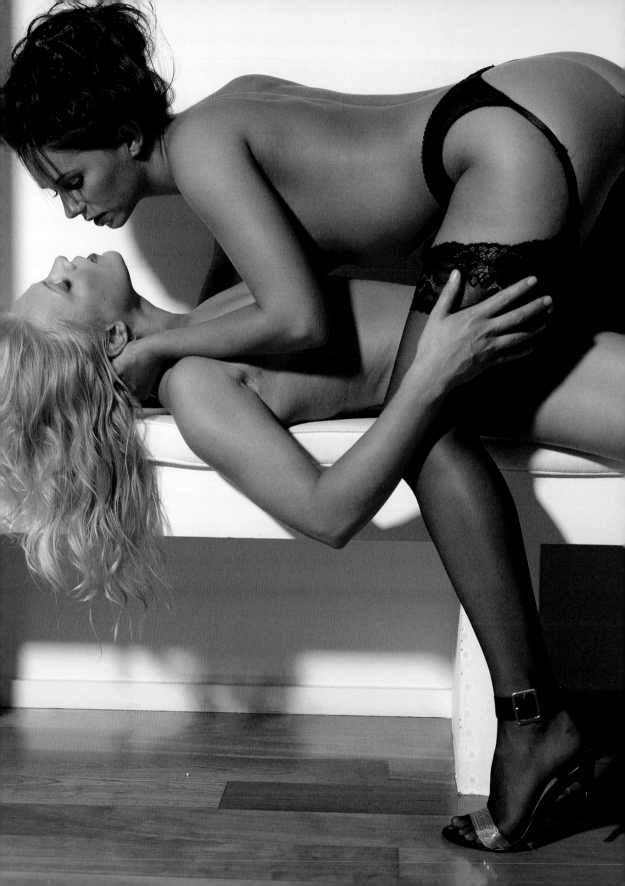

Bet you haven't tried...
Time to get *really* naughty

The world tends to divide into two types of couples: those who try anything and everything (S & M gear spilling out of their closets, serious-looking handcuffs dangling from the headboard) and those who don't really try anything at all (a half-forgotten vibrator in the nightstand drawer and a pair of naughty panties stuffed among Bridget Jones–style "Big Pants"). The majority of us fall into the latter

Watching her with a woman can be uncomfortable: **she's having *really* good sex (like, better than she ever has with you)** without an erect penis.

category—through sheer laziness, fear (scared to suggest it, scared people like our moms will find out), or romanticism (a perception that if you really love each other, you won't need any "false" stimulation—nonsense!). To prevent the inevitable decline in desire that affects almost all long-term couples, I'd suggest you take a step toward the middle of these two extremes. Create a new category of couples who experiment with interesting things, but aren't reliant on them to enjoy great sex. If you tried out some ideas from the previous chapter and enjoyed the results, you're ready to push the boat out a little farther into the erotic ocean. Again, don't panic! Despite the wonderfully risqué pictures in this feature, the ideas are adventurous but approached sensibly. I've started by giving you information about "risky" things you might be attracted to, then suggested a "wimp's way out": something naughty enough to "shock" your sexual system, but not so naughty it short-circuits the relationship.

SWINGING

Swingers are couples, usually in committed relationships, who like to have threesomes, foursomes, or moresomes with other couples. In the sex-crazy 70s, this was easy to achieve: simply invite all your neighbors over, serve large martinis along with the fondue and cheese-and-pineapple-on-toothpick appetizers (artistically stuck into an orange), and you'd all be pooling the car keys before the first joint got stubbed out. In today's moral climate, putting a hand up the

"A relationship is like a shark... it has to constantly move forward or it dies."

Woody Allen,
Annie Hall (1977)

Most **sex therapy** is aimed at making couples feel **comfortable sexually**. But new research suggests that **edginess, risk, and danger** are often needed to make **sex spectacular.**

sweater of nice Mrs. Johnson from next door, after your second glass of red wine, will probably end in handcuffs—but not quite the kind you were imagining. Most swingers these days meet through personal ads or via the Internet. Some couples keep it relatively private (well, as private as it can be), choosing only to play with one other couple at a time. Others attend swingers' parties or go to clubs, taking their pick from a broader selection. Generally, all couples arrive as a couple; most participate as a couple and leave as a couple. "Closed" swinging is when one partner chooses not to be around while their lover is having sex with others (highly sensible, I'd have thought); "open" swinging means both participate, and "soft" swinging means you'll "heavy pet" with people but draw the line at penetration. Not surprisingly, swinging comes with a hefty "try at your own risk" warning: you really do need to be a special type of person to cope with it. Most end up feeling jealous, and in lots of cases, motivation is lopsided. One partner wants to try it, the other goes along with it for fear of losing them if they don't. It can and does lead to split-ups, albeit interesting ones. I've interviewed at least four couples who have swapped with another couple—and stayed.

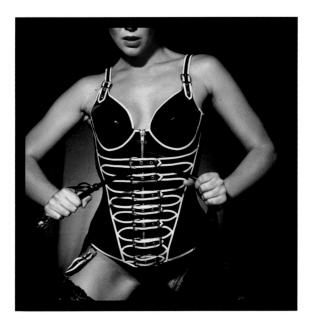

Wimp's way out:
Get the thrill of swinging without the downside by going to a swingers' club and watching but not participating. Choosing a club, planning what to wear, imagining all sorts of scenarios, finally turning up, giggly but excited—the anticipation of doing something terribly daring will already have injected more excitement into your relationship than you've seen since the new furniture store opened down the road. And you haven't even ventured inside yet! Once you do, you'll find that clubs are usually quite dark and anonymous, and it's relatively easy to hang back and observe without being asked to participate. Most have websites, so don't be

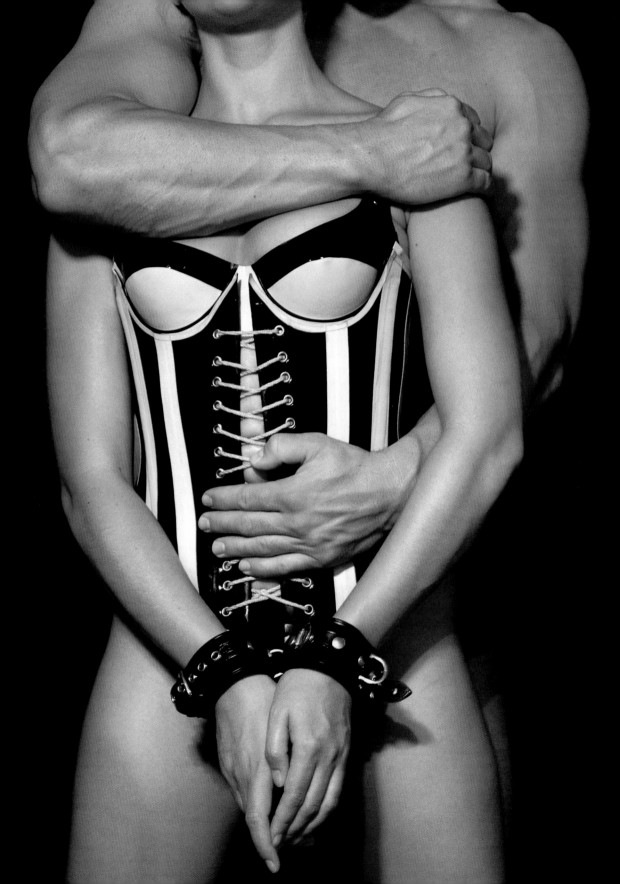

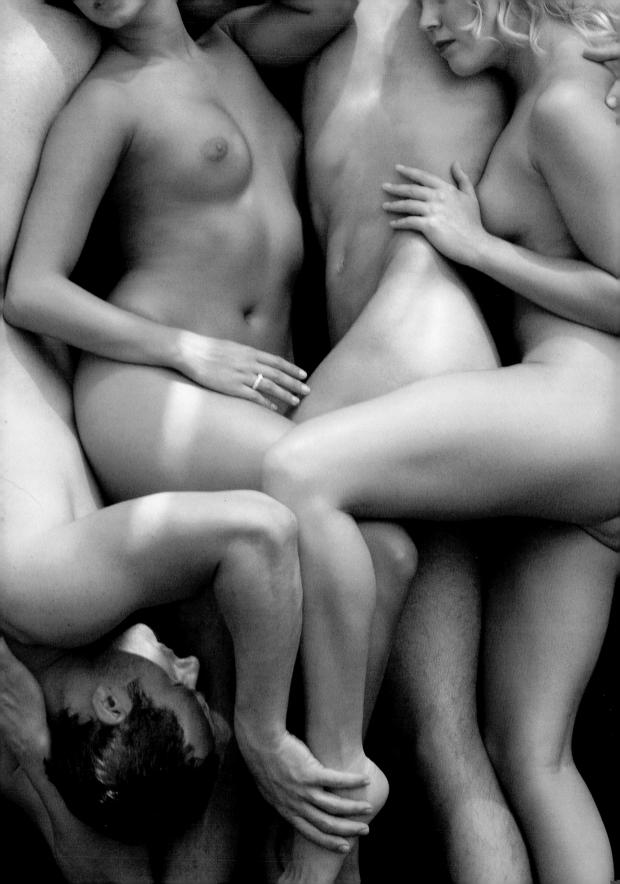

*A good
…d-fashioned orgy
…ed in Roman times
…se people were selfish
…ut their pleasure.
…ay, multiple bodies
…eans more people
to satisfy.*

…scared to email or call first to ask what "rules" there are (most clubs are cool with you just watching, but some aren't). Lots ask you to join as a member, but it's a legal formality—you can sign in as Elvis and Priscilla from Graceland for all they care. Bring lots of cash for the entrance fee and drinks, and aim to get there about two hours after it opens so there's plenty going on. Once inside, walk around and explore. There are usually several rooms and a general area that has porn playing. "Private rooms" are where couples can go to have sex. Sometimes there's a dance floor. Expect a lot of eyeing up and flirting, public displays of affection (and more), and a general air of seediness (which is, of course, why you're there). Stay as long as you're having fun, leave if you feel uncomfortable; don't drink too much.

WOMEN WITH WOMEN

…t's not just men who harbor secret fantasies of big-breasted blondes mud-wrestling; plenty of women are bi-curious. Wanting to experiment with the same sex isn't a problem if you're single and up for trying new things, but for long-term couples who've pledged monogamy, it poses a dilemma. You've promised not to sleep with anyone else—but does the rule still apply if it's someone of your own sex? Plenty of men respond to her initial suggestions of same-sex experimentation with delighted enthusiasm, a bit like they've just won the sexual lottery. But that's usually because (1) he assumes he will be allowed to watch and (2) he has a fixed script in his head of what will happen (the girls will kiss, fondle, and lick each other, putting on a fine show for him, but ultimately be bored with female flesh and beg him to join in and "properly" satisfy them). In reality, this often isn't the case. If she does allow him to watch (he's got about a 50/50 chance), the guy is often excluded as the girls get down to it, and he can't see as much as he thought (porn actors contort into ridiculous positions so the viewer can see the action). Then there's the risk that once she's batted for the home team, she'll want to stay on the bench with breasts. Some men "permit" their partner to experiment with women; others simply see it as sex with another person, which contravenes the relationship rules.

A safe way to indulge a same-sex fantasy is to visit a strip or lap-dancing club and let her flirt with the strippers and/or get a lap dance. No

Some couples plan to do daring things, then chicken out at the last minute. They're at the door of the swingers' club but find themselves heading to the nearest bar instead, hearts thudding and bits throbbing with the excitement of what *could* have happened. Even if you're not retracing your steps after the third drink, it doesn't mean you've "failed." The exercise has accomplished its purpose by simply pushing you out of your comfort zone.

If you and your partner are planning on watching rather than participating, make sure you time your entrance into the swingers' club carefully. Being one of the first couples to turn up is often disastrous! You feel self-conscious, the jaded regulars start licking their lips and drooling like a struggling dieter picking despondently at a salad, while friends dig in to a Sunday roast. Most swingers are friendly, but they may not be when misled.

longer just frequented by sad old drunks staring forlornly into their tumblers of scotch, strip and lap-dance bars now boast a clientele of hip young couples along with slightly tipsy groups of friends. Yes, the boisterous boys-night-out brigade is still there, ties askew and vomiting in the restroom, but if you choose carefully, they're in the minority. Women often get as much attention from strippers as the guys. If you want to make sure she does, load her up with the cash—the person doing the tipping gets all the attention. Some clubs have private peep booths where dancers masturbate or perform erotic acts (you pay by the minute); others have private VIP rooms where women play with sex toys and each other. Most strip clubs don't allow you to touch, and girls keep their distance, so if you want closer action, choose a lap-dance place. In some clubs they're totally naked, in others they're "clothed" (well, if you call thongs and wisps of next to nothing "clothes"). Ask if they have "couples' specials" where, in private, dancers perform simultaneous dances or spoil just one of you.

VOYEURISM AND "DOGGING"

A voyeur likes to watch other people have sex but doesn't want to join in (most are happy to masturbate). In a sense, we're all voyeurs: few of us would be able to resist watching people have sex if we knew we wouldn't get caught. True "peeping Toms,' however, actively search for spying opportunities (e.g., curtains left open) and are often unable to become aroused without "spying." Others pay sex workers to perform a private live show without feeling the need to participate, or indulge in what's called "dogging." Under the guise of taking the dog for a walk, they head to known "dogging" areas where exhibitionistic couples have sex in their car or singles masturbate.

Wimp's way out:

Peep booths perform the same purpose, without the risk of your being arrested (or shocking poor old Fido into an early doggie grave). Head toward the red light district in any city and you'll find them inside strip clubs and lots of adult book stores. Typically, you go inside, sit on a stool, put money or tokens into the meter, and a screen lifts or glass defogs to reveal a sex worker putting on a show behind glass. Sometimes you can request specific acts (for extra cash, of course).

"We are the most intensely excited when we are a little off-balance, uncertain, poised on the perilous edge between ecstasy and disaster."

Jack Morin,
The Erotic Mind

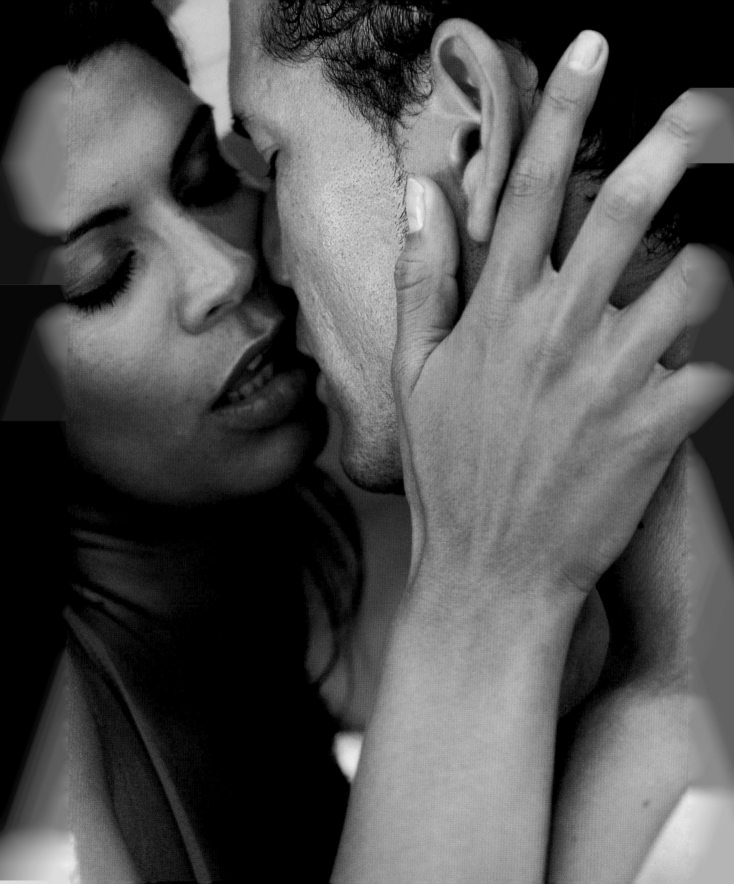

Thrills without spills
Raunchy new sex without the risks

I was (a naive) nineteen the first time someone asked me to do something "kinky." My fiancé (the first of three, before I actually followed through) tentatively suggested we turn to the porn channel while abroad and watch a "sexy movie" together.

Shocked, horrified, offended (and any other negative emotion you can think of), I drew myself up to full height (an impressive five-foot-five, to his six-foot-four) and said, outraged, "Absolutely not!" "No problem," he said, continuing to unpack, unconcerned. But I kept thinking about it. And thinking. And on the third day I said, "OK, let's give it a whirl," and, sexually, we never looked back. (OK, I looked forward, obviously, but never back.) My reaction is typical of most people. Feeling threatened and/or slightly shocked, we turn so moral and righteous, we'd make an 80-year-old nun look liberal. Persuading your partner to try new things sounds so simple... except it's often not. Here are some ideas on how to cope and what to do, on either side of the fence.

Sexploration: the rules

- **Talk** through exactly what will happen, being as specific as possible, so there are no surprises.
- **Set rules** and stick to them: how far are each of you prepared to go and under what circumstances?
- **Decide on a "safe word"** that means "Stop now." Make it something you're definitely not going to say accidentally.
- **Remember your relationship** is more important, at every moment, than the experience you're having. Constantly check in with each other.
- **Don't be afraid** to use your "safe word" to stop the experience if you feel upset. It doesn't mean you're prudish, just prudent.
- **If your partner gets upset**, stop everything immediately and go to their emotional rescue

OU want to try omething new, ey don't

emember, just because it turns you n, doesn't mean it's going to make hem shudder with delight: One person's vet dream is another's wet blanket.

e positive and confident when asking or what you want: If you make a big deal bout asking or look terrified once it's out of our mouth, they'll also think it's a big deal. Say confidently and casually and they're far more kely to agree. This is only possible if *you* truly elieve it's harmless fun. If you're secretly vorried it's dicey, slay your own personal emons first by finding out more about it.

e clear about what you want: Is this a ne-time experience or do you want it to be a egular part of your sex life? Most people can ope with doing "kinky" things consistently but regularly; few want to do it every single session.

alk it through: Asking someone to try omething new can make them feel insecure. hey think: "Why am I not enough anymore?" alking about the reasons why it appeals, actfully and laced with loads of sexual ompliments reassuring them they're still sexy, ften fixes the problem. Also ask if anything appened in their past that makes them not vant to do it now.

on't coerce or trick them: Threaten to eave or hint you'll get it elsewhere if they don't omply, and you deserve a slap—and not the ind you were after. Also, tying her up, saying Aha! Now I've got you!" and bringing in the all girl, isn't wise if you want to make that next vedding anniversary.

THEY want to try something new, you don't

- **Take it as a compliment:** They're showing trust and commitment by asking you, rather than taking the coward's way out and seeking it elsewhere.
- **Don't say no, say you'll think about it:** Educate yourself—read up about it, look on the Internet, then make a decision.
- **Understand why:** Ask your partner why it appeals to them. Let them reassure you it doesn't mean you don't turn them on anymore, they're simply craving variety.
- **Take baby steps:** If your partner wants to try phone sex with a professional, for instance, go online and talk dirty in a chatroom. Only when you feel you're ready, move on.
- **Consider doing it for them:** If it's something they're desperate to try and you're not completely adverse to it, why not make their day? Making them as happy as an ex-smoker who's just been told cigarettes are actually good for them, could be enough of a reward. And seeing them turned on can often turn you on.
- **Consider doing it for you:** What can you get out of it? Being spanked or tied up, for instance, means you get to lie back and do nothing.
- **Strike up a deal:** There's nothing wrong with sexual bartering if it's done in a spirited, friendly fashion.
- **Risk the unfamiliar:** Remember this mantra: If you keep doing what you've always done, you'll keep getting what you've always gotten. If your love life rates as "content," take a risk.

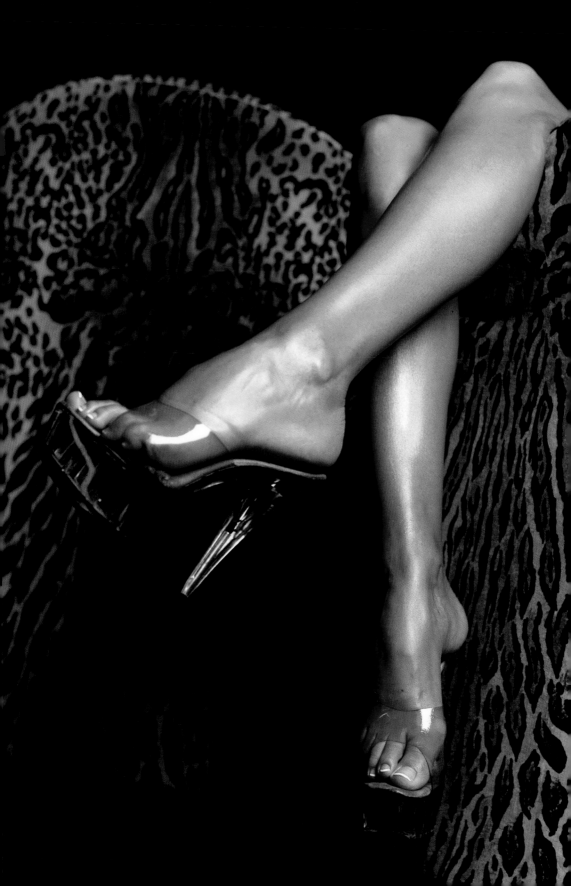

Lashings of lust
Take a tip (not just the whip) from S & M

Being into S & M now is like being gay 25 years ago. Bondage (tie-up games) jumped the fence between kinky and commonplace some time ago, spanking is currently straddling it, and S & M is pawing at the ground, poised to take a flying leap, but hasn't landed yet. Back in 1980, being gay was accepted by the young and open-minded but still raised eyebrows and huffs and puffs in others. S & M is equally borderline: true devotees are still considered "weird" and unsavory by the great

The dominant will stop at nothing to possess you... but if they ask you to lick the toilet clean with your tongue, feel free to tell them to get lost!

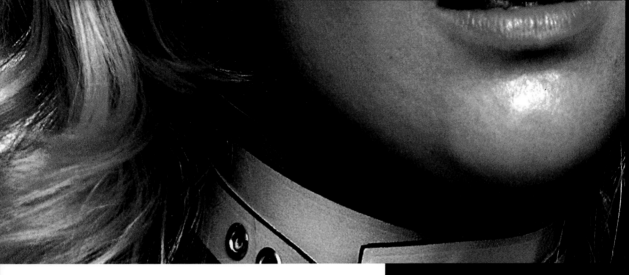

comfort them afterward. The dominant person usually has a name—"Master," "Mr.," "Mistress," "Ma'am"—that denotes authority. You can add their real name after (Mistress Tracey, for instance—I like that!). The dominant chooses the submissive's name—and at the mention of it, they must obey! Some people name their genitals, then use it as code ("Violet wants you to talk to her'"), others find they can't master that part without laughing.

Pitch it right

If you're the dominant, then wimpy, soft, girly little voices won't do. Pitch your voice deeper than usual; speak loudly and in staccato sentences like "Get me that." "Would you mind?", "Please," and "Thank you" are banned. (Your great aunt might be horrified, but your partner will shiver with pleasure!) Maintain eye contact, move quickly, and make "big" gestures. Stand with your hands on your hips, don't smile, hold your head high. Submissives should drop their eyes, make themselves "small," keep their head bowed, and act exaggeratedly grateful for any small mercies.

What do I do next?

You're limited only by your imagination. If you're struggling for ideas, try these: • masturbate just out of reach • blindfold them • spank them • remind them they're helpless and tell them what you're going to do to them • alternate fast sex with slow, torturous sex • use sex toys on them • tie them up • make them stand, hands bound, while you go about your business • order them to wear particular clothes or sit in a certain way • forbid them to climax • shave their genitals • use hot and cold sensations (ice cubes, warm coffee).

The rules

- **Don't use a discipline session to work out a problem** (i.e., if you really are angry about something, strangely, this isn't the way to vent it).

- **Have a "safe word"**—a word both of you know means "Stop right now." Always, always stop when it's uttered, without demanding an explanation first.

- Three words to keep in mind: **safe, sane, and consensual.**

- **Keep it private**—it's not for entertaining your friends with—and don't mock each other once the scenario is over.

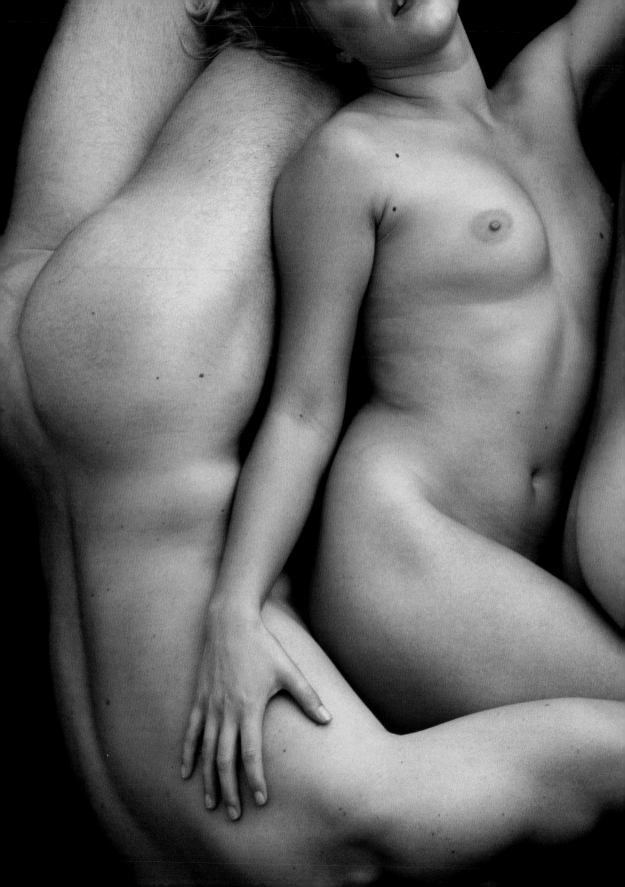

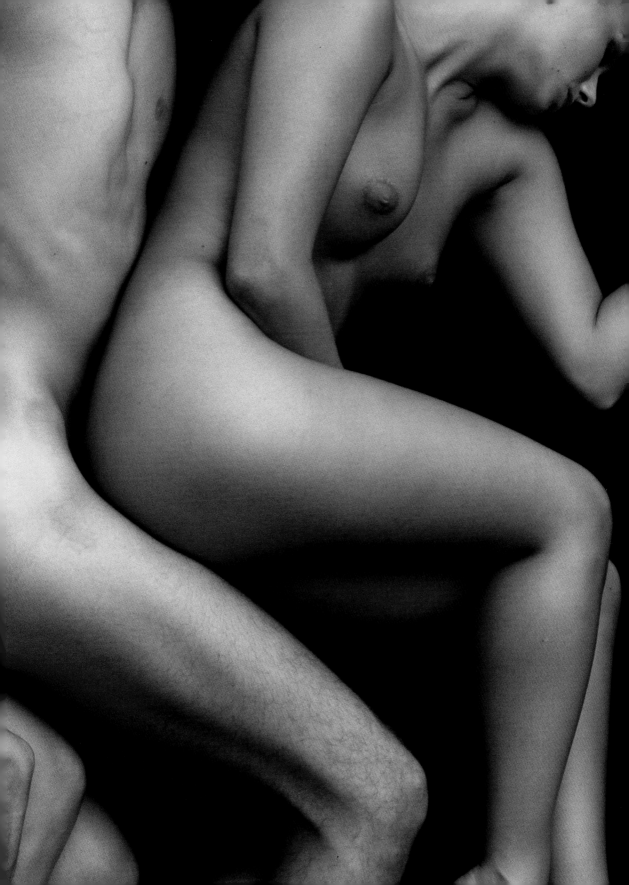

Threesomes
Twice the fun or asking for trouble?

Having a threesome pretty much always tops the most popular fantasy list—particularly for men. And although I'm biased against anything that involves inviting extra bodies into the bed (very few committed couples manage to negotiate these scenarios successfully), I can see the appeal.

Two men, both indulging my every need simultaneously—I mean, hello! Who wouldn't enjoy that? If you want to experiment with the same sex, a three-way makes it seem less threatening, and it appears to solve the need for new flesh without lying or going behind your partner's back. These are all good, sound reasons for experimenting. And if you're single or in a casual relationship that you don't mind risking, go for it (though still please read the advice below).

If you're in a long-term, committed relationship, however, be warned: indulging this fantasy may not turn out to be the exotic, erotic adventure you'd imagined. Jealousy is a huge problem (feeling left out, thinking your partner prefers the other person), with nasty surprises running a close second. Seeing your partner's penis disappear down the throat of a stranger as his eyes roll back in bliss, may not be quite the turn-on you thought it would be. Plenty of females freak when it suddenly dawns on them they won't be the only one playing with the male newcomer, and kissing (on the surface the most innocent activity of all) is the cause of much horrendous fallout. Deciding exactly what will happen beforehand helps, but the reality is often still quite shocking. Yes, there are couples who have three-ways regularly and swear it's enhanced rather than damaged their relationship. But they're the exception rather than the rule, and quite frankly, there are so many other deliciously naughty but safe suggestions in this book, I'd much rather you didn't take the risk. If, however, after much consideration, you decide to go ahead, I've provided a few guidelines. Along with these are some less risky alternatives to get the thrill of a three-way, without the potential pitfalls.

IF YOU DECIDE TO DO IT:
• **Be careful who you approach.** Sexy friends, colleagues, or acquaintances may seem like a good idea—but not so inspired when they're horrified by your suggestion (even the most sexually liberated often pale when it comes to coming with friends—it seems wrong somehow), it all goes horribly wrong, and/or you've lost a great friendship. Instead, consider my suggestions (see right) of safer ways to create a threesome, go to sex-themed parties (fetish or swingers' parties, etc.) where people are more open to the suggestion, or answer or place an ad in a newspaper or on a website. If it were me, I'd probably have one while overseas, away from prying eyes and pervy neighbors.

- **Always, always practice safe sex.**
- **Never have a threesome unless both of you want one.** Doing it because your partner has threatened to leave if you don't agree, is plain ridiculous. Ditch your partner instead—and good riddance to anyone who uses emotional blackmail.
- **Never surprise** your partner with a threesome.
- **Make rules on what is and isn't allowed.** Decide who can do what, to whom beforehand.
- **Do only the things that turn you on** and make you both feel good.
- **Don't take being left out personally.**
- **Pay your partner more attention** than the third person.
- **Stop if you become upset.** Use code words only you two understand: "red" (stop), "green" (having fun), "orange" (not sure but want to keep going). (The third person may think you're nuts, but I'm more worried about keeping you two happy).
- **Pile on the compliments** afterward (they were more attractive/sexier than the third person).

SAFER WAYS TO PLAY

- **Role-play it instead** by inviting vibrators and dildos into your bed, along with a blindfold. It feels like you're making love with more than one person, without actually doing it. You can perform imaginary fellatio to a third party on a vibrator.
- **Watch erotic same-sex videos** If he wants two women, watch lesbian porn (you're not going to be starved for choice!). If she craves two men, rent a DVD with a threesome theme. Mimic the action— you might be surprised how realistic it can feel.

A sexy alternative

Another way to capture the sense of this fantasy is to have phone sex with a professional. Yes, she probably will be doing the ironing in her jogging pants, phone tucked under her chin, but you'd never guess it. Professional phone sex workers spend all day and night telling stories, listening to fantasies, and making callers climax through words— most of them are damn good at their job!

If you've got a speaker phone, use it. That way no one's left out and you both have the freedom to caress and lick each other as you're listening to her talk. Or try one partner talking, while the other does whatever the girl on the end of the phone is suggesting. (If you can't hear her, get your partner to repeat out loud what she's saying.) If she agrees and you can put her on speaker phone, you can get her to take the two of you through a particularly naughty sex session, directing your every move. Or if you've got two phones, you can both listen separately and masturbate.

A few words of warning: don't use work or a friend's phones to call and, if you're worried, ask how it will appear on your phone bill. (It's unlikely they're doing business as "Extremely Dirty Phone Sex" but check anyway.) When you call to reserve the session, tell them what sort of fantasy you want to indulge.

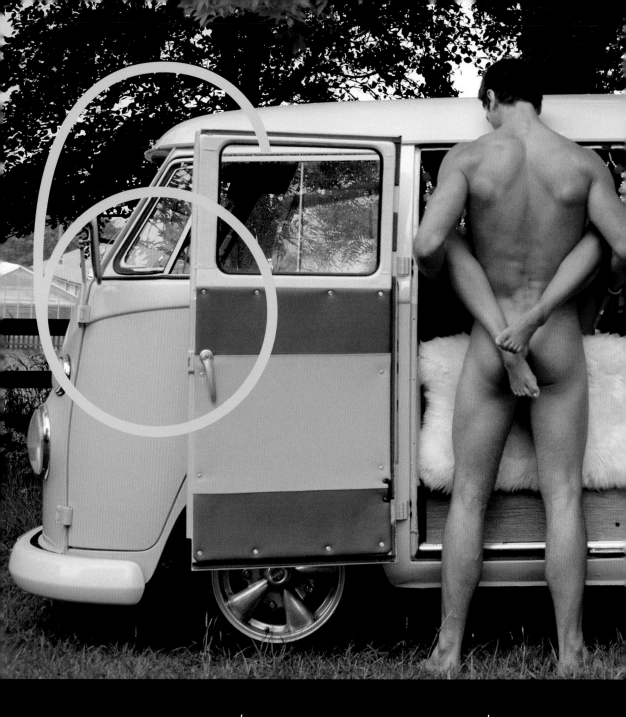

Tantric, Tao, the Kama Sutra and how spiritual sex can satisfy more than just your body. If you want sex with soul, you might just find it here.

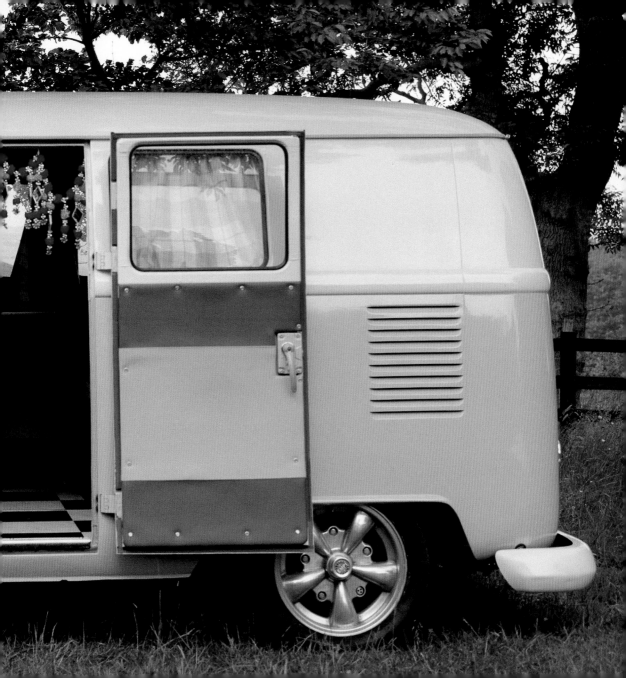

Grassroots sex

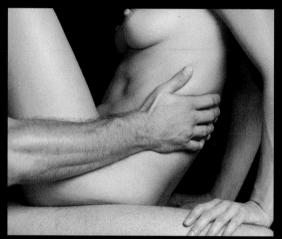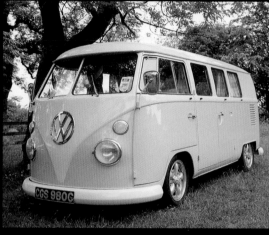

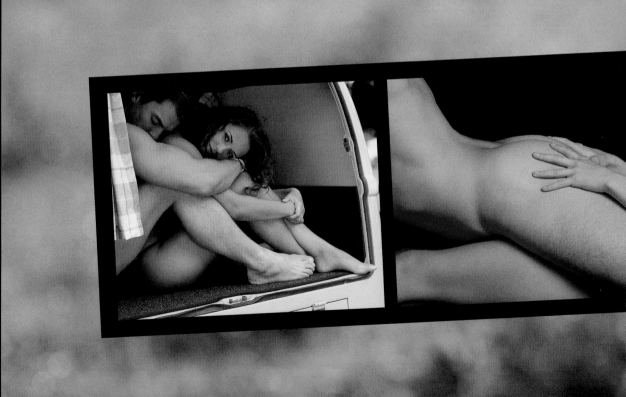

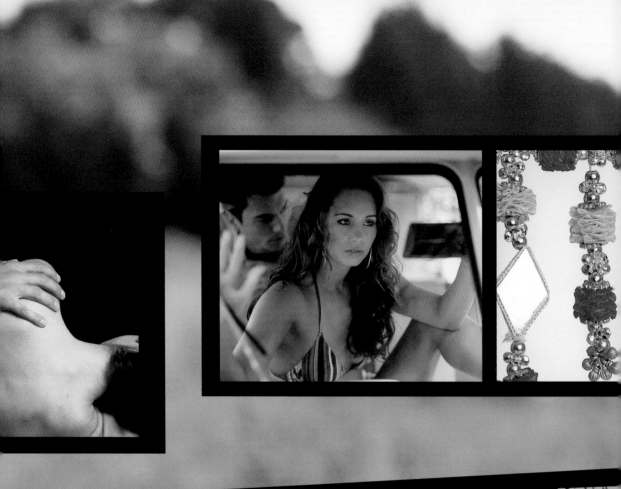
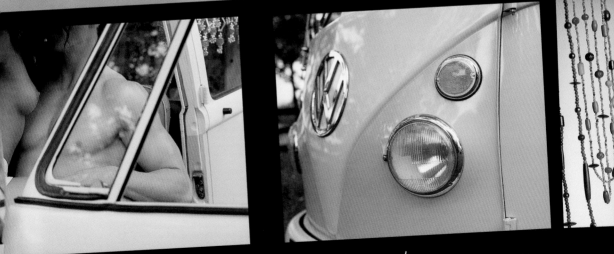

Get an Eastern edge with sex that encourages intimacy, togetherness, and sensual exploration.

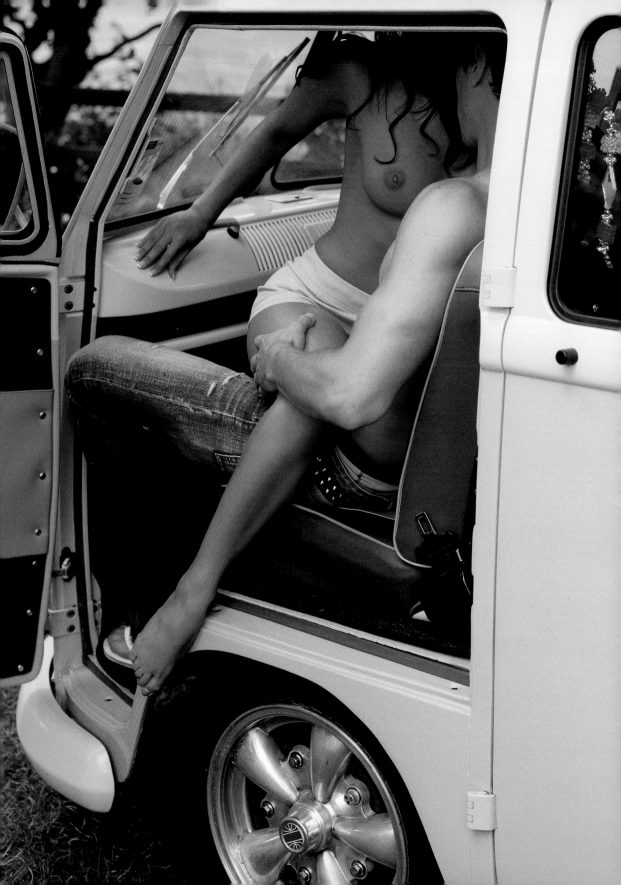

Cosmic connection
How to put the *Ahhh!* into Om

I have to be honest and say I initially approached the topic of spiritual sex with great skepticism. It might well be based on concepts and principles drawn from musty, ancient texts (which makes us automatically assume the content is wise), but let's all be honest here: some of it really is a bunch of BS. Like, does anyone really "get down on all fours and pretend to be lions roaring at one another"? Please, God, tell me no. While I can think of some very good reasons to get down on all fours, pretending to be a lion isn't one of them.

It's not a myth that **Tantric sex** can go on for one to two hours, but the jury's still out on whether **longer** sex equals more **enjoyable sex.**

I'm also not terribly impressed by claims that loss of semen weakens a man and shortens his life. If this is true, how come Hugh Hefner is still alive? A spiritual sex fan, I wasn't! Until I started reading in earnest and... if you can get past the let's-all-pretend-we're-little-flowers-growing-in-the-earth stuff, there's actually some damn good, sound advice mixed in there. I emerged from the research pleasantly surprised—and, dare I say, a tad converted! (Academic research, not practical stuff, by the way—sadly, I really don't lie around instantly testing out every theory with a never-ending stream of gorgeous men!)

Now, before I attempt to pass on what I think are the best parts, I must point out I'm not even going to attempt to summarize the true spiritual meanings and intellectual theories behind my discoveries. Fascinating as it is, the sex part of the *Kama Sutra* is in fact just one book in a series of seven, and to truly embrace and understand Tantra takes a lifetime. Besides, we're different creatures than we were back

Why you might like it
• Lots of the mushy stuff (e.g., hands on hearts, synchronizing breathing) can make people feel more secure.
• It's creative and new.
• Couples are encouraged to live in the moment, take time out, and watch stress levels.
• There's no rush to orgasm.
• You're told to make a sacred space; clean sheets and scented candles make a nice change from dog hair and toast crumbs.

then. Our lifestyles, beliefs, and values have changed, so some of the cultural and spiritual beliefs could be hard to relate to. Instead, I'm going to focus on practical sex tips or lessons we can learn. If you like what you're reading and think you'd like to explore more, put down that bowl of lentils and get onto the Net or into a bookstore to choose from lots of great books on the subject of spiritual sex. This is a mere "taster" of what to expect from each—turn to page 146 if you'd like to try out some Tao or Tantric techniques; see page 150 for Kama Sutra–style positions.

Does anyone really **"get down on all fours and pretend to be lions roaring at one another"?** Please, God, tell me no.

TANTRA
What is it? It's an Eastern science that emerged out of a rebellion against a Hindu belief that suggested sex was a no-no if you wanted "spiritual enlightenment." It's been around since the seventh century and honors the sacred union of the male and female energies that create life. Shiva, the male Hindu god, is the embodiment of pure consciousness; and Shakti, the female, is the embodiment of pure energy.

The basic principles: Sex is slowed down. There's gradual, controlled thrusting, rather than the usual frenetic free-for-all. This enables women to use learned techniques like vaginal tensing and flexing—a fancy version of pelvic floor exercises. (It's not a myth Tantric sex can go on for one or two hours, by the way, but the jury's still out on whether longer sex sessions lead to more enjoyable sex.) Tantra also teaches you how to stay in the moment. If you're the type to drift off while your partner's still gamely thrusting away ("When will I go to the gym tomorrow?"), the "connecting" exercises could be useful. Traditional sex therapy encourages people to lose themselves in the experience, whereas Tantra is all about staying fully aware and present. Breathing exercises are designed to improve sexual tone, prolong intercourse, and can help men who have premature ejaculation.

Lessons to learn
- It encourages couples to stop being time- or orgasm-focused.
- Tantric techniques involve the heart as well as other parts.
- There's no place in Tantra for lovers to be selfish— it's all about giving.

spiritual sex is perfect for older men who may take longer to become aroused. As the saying goes, "What young men want to do all night, takes older men all night to do."

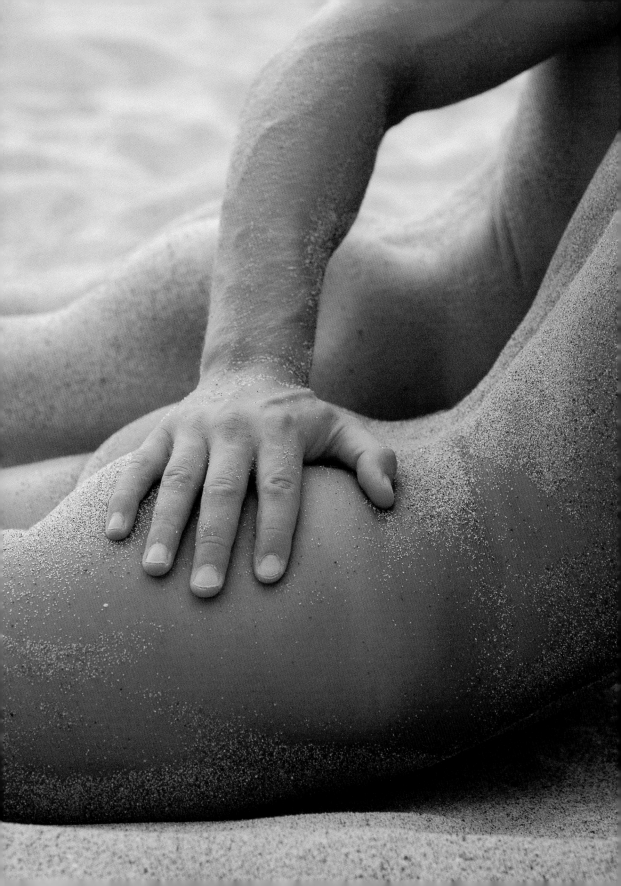

You're taught to let go of body judgments. "Fat days"
don't exist because you learn to love all of you.
(Or because you look like the girl in this photo.)

- Men are encouraged to prolong lovemaking (the old "retain your semen" thing again), which buys into the myth that women climax through penetration.
- Rituals are important. Some people love this aspect, others hate having to go through long, complicated processes just to get some action.
- Tantra often refers to mixing of body fluids ("nectar" or "love juices"). If you're not having monogamous sex, mixing is about as sensible as lying in the middle of a freeway during rush hour. Safe sex and condoms aren't figured in.

Tantric sex teaches you how to stay in the moment. So if you're the type of person who drifts off while **your partner** is still gamely **thrusting away**, it could be very useful...

KAMA SUTRA

What is it? It's an ancient sex manual written between the third and fifth centuries. There are actually seven books in total, though only the second is devoted purely to sex. (Worth wading through the others, however, if you'd like to know how to break into a harem or how to conduct an affair successfully!) The *Kama Sutra* is much, much more than just acrobatic positions for intercourse, though most modern interpretations focus almost exclusively on this. Ironically, the suspected author of the sex book (Vatsyayana) was a lifelong celibate.

The basic principles: Interestingly, all the complex seduction and sexual techniques actually aren't aimed at couples in love. If you love each other, all you need to do is "let yourself go and be led by instinct." (Oh, really?) The techniques are designed to help you achieve this state. Some positions seem yoga-like because they're designed to facilitate meditation as a couple. They're also intended to allow you to have sex for one or two hours with minimal movement needed. During this time, you will exchange vital energies—or fall asleep. (My money's on the latter.)

Modern manuals?
Originally, ancient sex manuals like the *Kama Sutra* and *The Perfumed Garden* were hidden from women— it was the man's job to learn how to pleasure his woman. Despite the off-putting sexist connotations, both texts are refreshingly open about topics we've since become uptight about. Both provide early examples of tasteful pornography and encourage masturbating in front of each other.

Lessons to learn

- It recognized female orgasm in a time when others thought there was no such thing.
- It recommends the man ensures she climaxes before he does.
- Sexual boredom and monotony are seen as the reason why couples split up.
- It's common in India for men to be encouraged to read the *Kama Sutra* before marrying. (If the West instituted this type of premarital sex research, I think affairs and divorce rates would fall dramatically!)

Not so sure

- A man and woman live as one single body and soul. Independent types and commitment-phobes would run screaming for the hills.
- Those one- to two-hour sessions... sorry to carp, but who's got time?
- Some of the positions require rubber limbs and plasticine penises.

According to the Kinsey report, 15–20 percent of young men are capable of repeated orgasm in a limited period of time. 14 percent of females clock up multiple orgasms regularly.

TAOISM

What is it? The Tao is a book written in the sixth century that talks about the yin (female) and the yang (male) and the flow of energy between them. This energy is called ch'i and it's the same life force that flows in the human body. Couples achieve harmony by learning how to live within the flux of changing energy.

The basic principles: Taoism recognized that men can have multiple orgasms because orgasm and ejaculation are two separate processes. (Ejaculation is simply the series of contractions that pumps the semen out; the feeling of orgasm happens in the brain.) Using long, involved "Sting-like" processes, men are taught to train their brain and body to separate orgasm from ejaculation. There's a focus on lots of foreplay and nine types of thrusting to try—the aim being to achieve 81 thrusts (one set of nine of each type)!

Lessons to learn

- It recognizes that male desire is easier to ignite and quick to burn out, while female arousal takes longer but tends to last longer.
- There's an emphasis on slow, prolonged foreplay with lots of finger and mouth action for her.

Not so sure

- Who's going to keep count until you get to 81?
- Ejaculation is permitted only when necessary. Call my male friends old-fashioned, but none thought this was a good thing.
- Separating orgasm from ejaculation is something I've read lots about, but I've never met a man who's actually mastered it. Most women aren't that bothered and would probably be highly suspicious, rather than in raptures, of an apparent orgasm without any evidence (men fake it, too).
- One suggested method for stopping orgasm is for him to "gnash his teeth." This, I suspect, would not be terribly sexy for her.

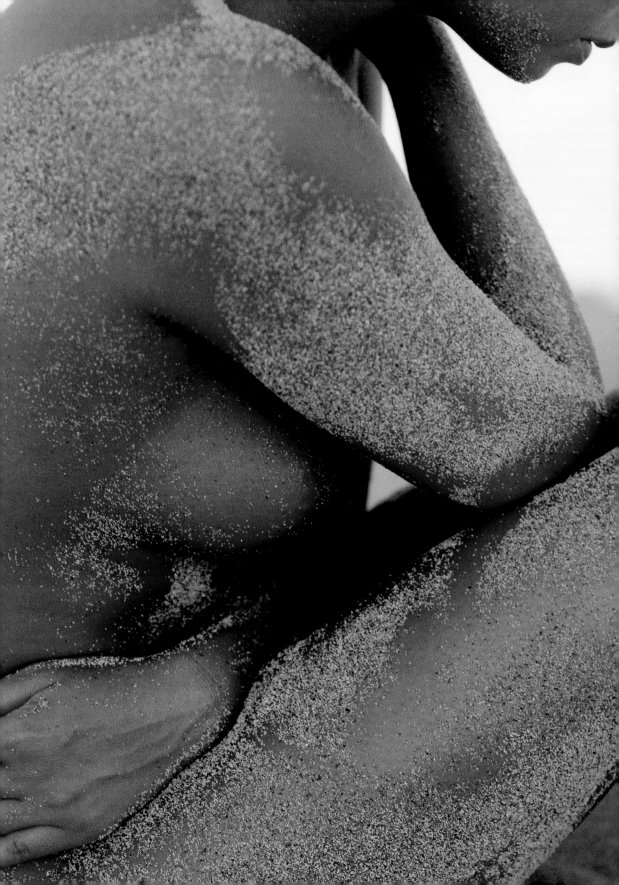

Take a test drive
Tao and Tantric techniques to try

TO HAVE A FULL-BODY ORGASM

Forget clitoral, vaginal, G-spot, or multiple, the full-body orgasm supposedly makes all the competition pale in comparison. We're talking hot dogs versus filet mignon, thrift-store hand-me-downs versus designer clothes... well, according to a Tantrika (someone who's into Tantra), anyway. They claim that by learning certain Tantric techniques, you can not only flood your entire body with orgasmic sensations, you can stay there for minutes or over an hour. You accomplish this by opening your "chakras"—the body's energy centers. These are located at the base of the spine, stomach, genitals, throat, forehead, and crown of the head.

Techniques that could help get you one

- **Start with massage:** Her massage concentrates on the lower back, spine, and the inside surface of her arms and legs. His focuses on the central area of the feet, which indirectly stimulates the liver (which controls and releases blood needed for erection).
- **Get the balance right:** Taoists encourage men to absorb the woman's fluids. It's called "the great liberation of the three peaks." (Yes, really.) In non-Taoist terms, this basically means he must lick her lips and tongue, her breasts, and her genitals. Secretions from these parts are supposedly fabulous for his health—chances are she won't argue otherwise.
- **Read the signs:** Spiritualists believe it's possible for both of you to achieve "supreme pleasure" if the man pays attention to five significant signs of female desire. (In case you hadn't noticed, a lot of spiritual sex is focused on the woman, which could possibly explain my warming enthusiasm!) This is what you're looking for: 1. When she blushes and her body temperature rises, she's in the mood for "tender play." 2. When her nipples harden and small drops of sweat appear around her nose, she's ready to be penetrated. 3. If her throat or lips seem dry, she wants faster and deeper thrusts. 4. When her lubrication turns "slippery," he should move into the "deep explosion" (keep thrusting and don't stop) and squeeze his body against hers, each time with "more insistence." 5. When he spots secretions of a thick fluid on her thighs, she's reached the "high tide" of orgasmic explosion. Sadly for him, he's forced to keep wading in the shallow end. Instead of being able to let go and orgasm after all that hard work, he's advised to immediately begin his breathing exercises to postpone ejaculation for as long as possible. The two of you then switch into various intercourse positions, in search of the infamous "supreme pleasure." The whole thing sounds (and is) both pleasurable and a pain in the ass. Speaking of which, by the way, there's more than one technique involving anal penetration for him in spiritual sex, the rectum being the home of the male "G-spot" (prostate gland).

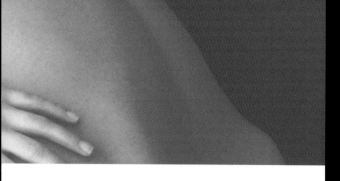

TO DELAY EJACULATION

- **Find the Million Dollar Point:** One of the oldest Taoist techniques involves pressing the "Million Dollar Point" while he contracts his PC muscle (the one you'd use to stop yourself from urinating). This helps delay ejaculation by interrupting the ejaculatory reflex. This technique is best mastered by him initially. Ideally, guys, you'd push your finger inside your anus, up to the first joint, searching for a small indentation. The squeamish could try to find it by pressing it externally through the perineum (the area between the testicles and anus).
- **Do a Finger Lock:** When you're hovering close to a spill-the-seed moment, press the three middle fingers of your strongest hand into the Million Dollar Point, hard enough to stop the flow of semen. (Do it externally, pushing on the perineum.) You're basically pushing your middle finger against the urethral tube, which swells when close to ejaculation, making it easier to find. The other fingers press on each side of the tube to hold it in place. Once you've done this, contract your PC muscle and "draw" your orgasmic energy up to the spine and to your brain. (Yes, you possibly will take a few attempts to get the hang of that last part.) Hold your fingers in place until the contractions and pumping stop completely. If you're a very good boy and practice a LOT, you eventually can rely purely on a mind technique called "the big draw" to stop ejaculation. You will, understandably, lose your erection after doing the Finger Lock. But that's sort of the point, and it will return with a vengeance before you can say, "Oops! Time to do *another* Finger Lock."

A sampler of the other stuff

- **Mantras** are spoken or chanted during Tantric sex, the most famous and common one being *om mani padme hum. Mani* means "thunderbolt" (referring to his penis), *padme* means "lotus" (vagina), and *hum* is the highest form of enlightenment. Tantrikas chant to awaken sexual energy and to mimic the energy vibration of the universe.

- **The five M's or *pancamakara*** appears, on the surface, to be hedonistic heaven—a feast followed by an orgy (now we're talking!). The first four involve eating and drinking aphrodisiacs. The fifth is *maithuna*—ritualistic sex that allows you to experience "higher" pleasure while your body's still digesting the physical type. If you were a man who lived in (glorious) times past, you might have had *maithuna* with over 100 women a night. The point of this, however, wasn't to boast to your friends later, but to surpass mortal pleasure and reach a form of connection through performing specific ritualistic sex. People moved very little during these acts, possibly because the vaginal secretion was collected from the woman's genitals afterward and mixed with a bowl of water. This was offered to the gods; later, the man drank the water, completing the circle.

To keep things simple, try these: For harmonious sex, press similar body parts together—lips to lips, hands to hands, genitals to genitals. For excitement and stimulation, press dissimilar body parts together—mouth to genitals, mouth to breast, penis to anus, etc.

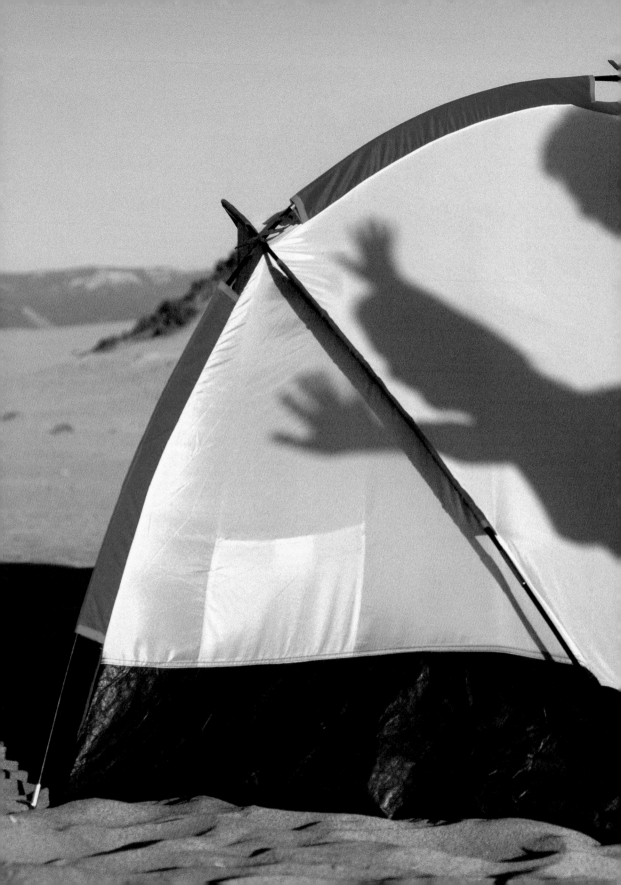

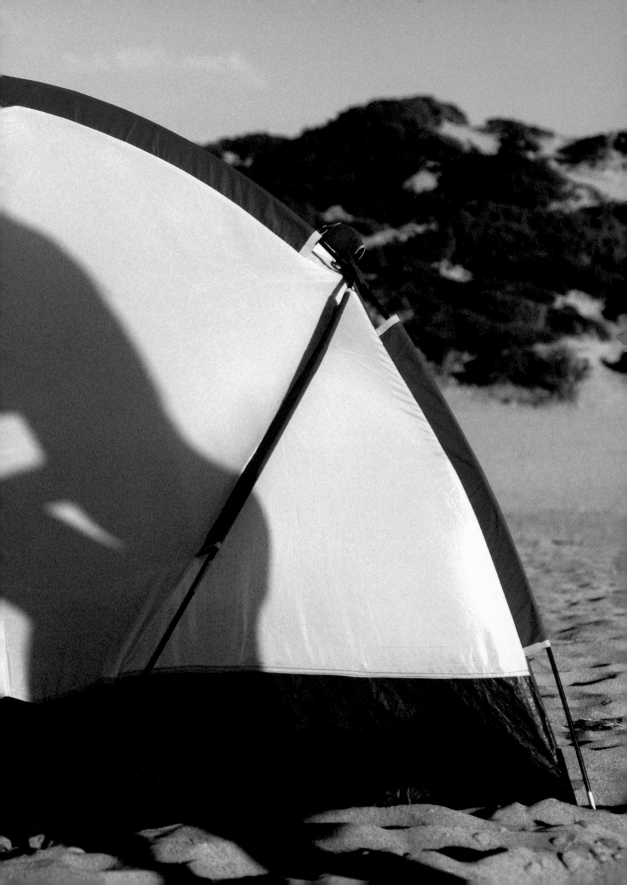

The 10 all-time-best show-off sex positions

1

LEGGING IT

Inspired by the *Kama Sutra*, this position is suitable for the "highest congress"—meaning the vagina is fully open to allow for maximum penetration. She is fully exposed, showing her "wet and longing" parts to her partner, which can be one hell of a turn-on for both of you. He has a great view, watching his penis move in and out. You can't kiss because your faces can't get close, which ups the erotic tension and makes you concentrate solely on penetration.

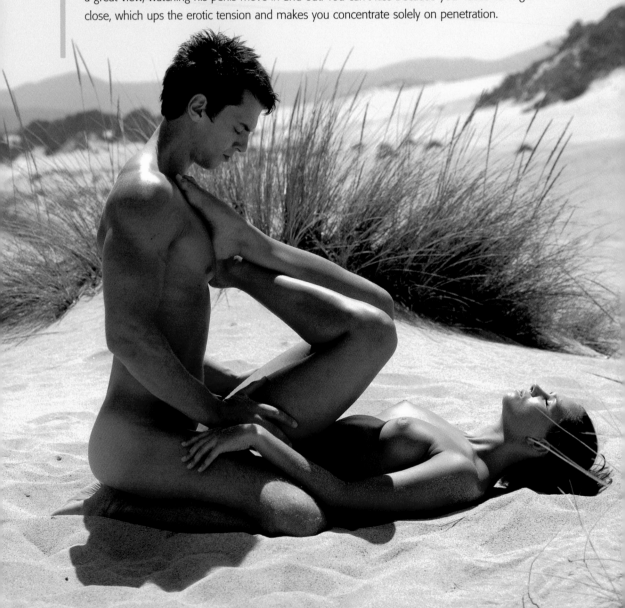

2

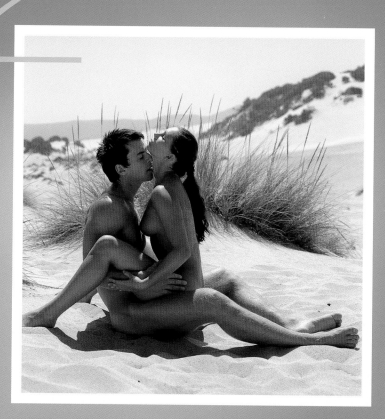

THE TANTRIC MELT

A version of a Tantric sitting posture, this ensures you'll "be as one" by "dissolving" into each other. Eye contact combined with close torsos makes it intimate, and you can practice synchronizing your breath (if it appeals!). Interestingly, this pose puts both of you in a power position. She's on top, so can control the rhythm, speed, and depth of thrusting, but she's also effectively sitting in his lap, which is a traditionally submissive female pose. If she sat higher and rested her thighs in the crook of his elbow, he could lift her, taking complete control.

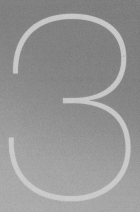

3

SIDE STRADDLE

A pose with significance, the shape of this pose replicates a specific pattern the ancient Chinese used when fusing two pieces of jade together. She lies on her side, bending one leg at the knee and drawing it upward. He kneels behind her, straddling her side-on, and entering her at a sideways angle, holding her shoulder to keep her in place. It's precise positioning, which gets you both in the mood for controlled, disciplined sex.

A **rival to the *Kama Sutra*,** *The Perfumed Garden* details **six movements**—like "bucket in the well"—to try during **intercourse.**

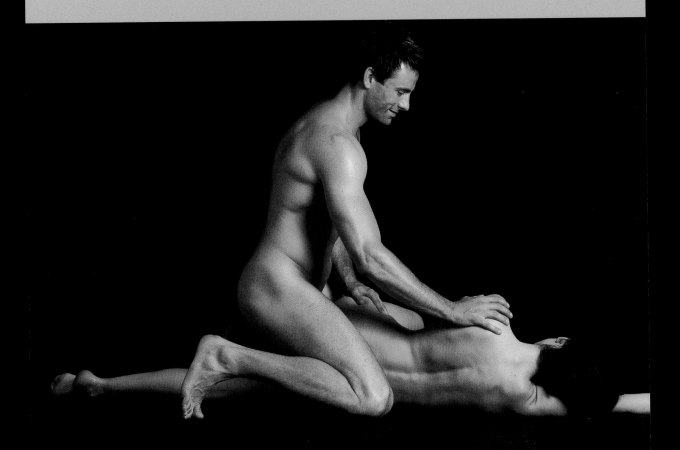

4

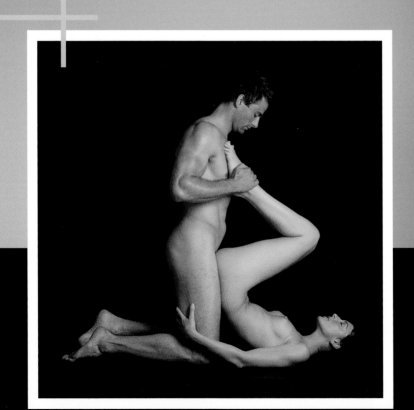

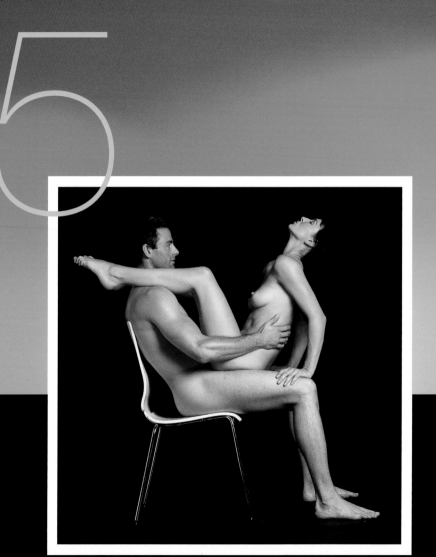

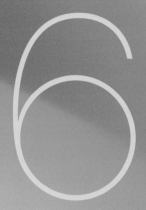

TOPSY TURVY

Who said the missionary position is boring?! Spin it around for a sensational twist. If he's adventurous, he'll enter in the traditional position (heads on the same end) and slowly spin until he's facing the opposite way. The more sensible penetrate while in position (and yes, it is difficult). She'll like it because her clitoris and labia are in contact with his pelvis, adding much-needed pressure. If he's into anal stimulation, she's in the perfect place to penetrate with a well-lubricated finger. If she's into toe-sucking, this is the position for you!

The **less adventurous** can accomplish **"Balanced Babe"** by getting her to sit up, lean forward, and **put her feet on the floor.**

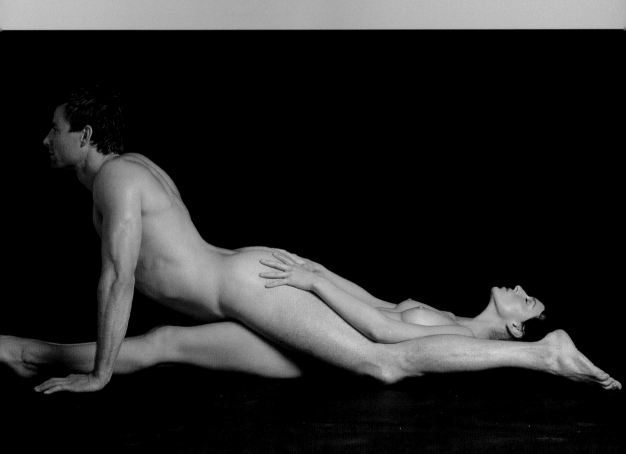

7

THE CAVE

The *Kama Sutra* rather charmingly extols the virtues of positions like this because she offers her "red cave" for him to admire before penetration. Not for girls who find touching their toes a challenge; rubbery, supple, s-t-r-e-t-c-h-e-d limbs are a necessity. Normal thrusting is impossible; instead, rock in a seesaw motion. With legs closed, the vaginal canal becomes invitingly narrow; she spreads her legs for wider access and deeper penetration.

The Cave is great for men with short penises because it **raises, tilts, and exposes** the vulva, making it **feel better** for both of you.

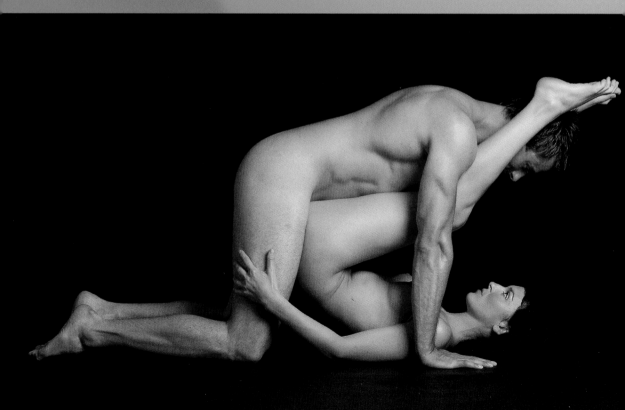

8

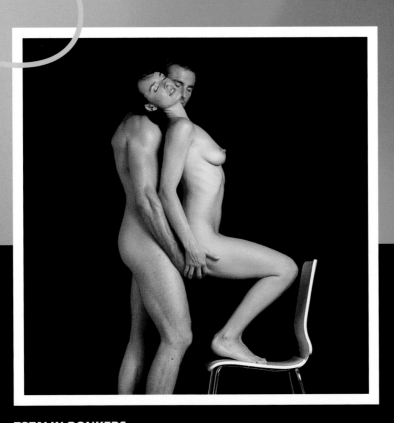

TOTALLY BONKERS

This is the position you'd dearly love your partner's gorgeous ex to catch you in. "Advanced" isn't the word for it; "bonkers" probably is. If you're using a chair, for God's sake, make sure it's wedged firmly up against a wall. (A very hard bed can also work.) She leans her shoulders back against his chest as he penetrates, tipping her bottom upward toward him to make penetration possible. If he keeps slipping out (and he will), she spreads her legs wider and tips her bottom up even higher. This has all the trademarks of *Kama Sutra*—it looks impractical, but if he's strong and she's supple, it is possible. Just.

9

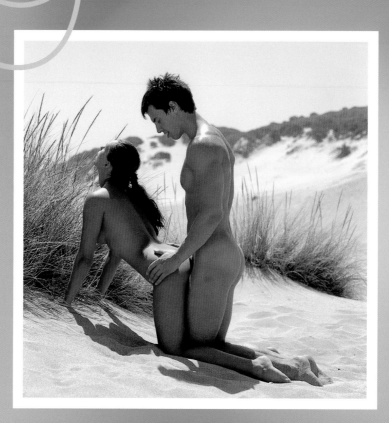

THE BULL

Erotic sculptures of "the man mounting the woman like a bull" can be found in Hindu temples. Tantra doesn't shy from animalistic sex, and acting out the postures of animals is seen as liberating for both sexes. This typical rear-entry position means she "surrenders" to him completely... but she can lean backward or forward to alter the angle of the vagina, so is still (semi) in control. It allows both to fantasize, and he can thrust deeply, with a fabulous view of her buttocks thrown in for good measure!

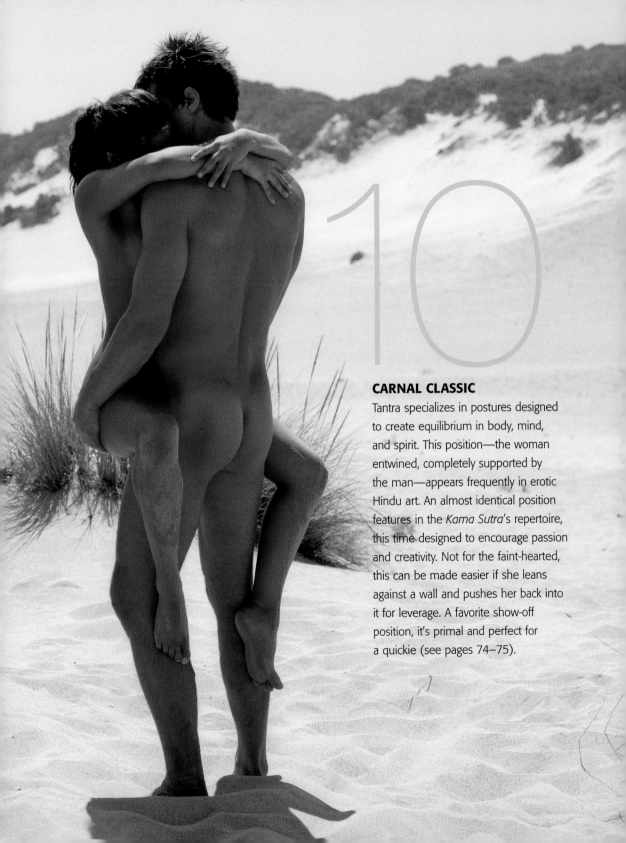

10

CARNAL CLASSIC

Tantra specializes in postures designed to create equilibrium in body, mind, and spirit. This position—the woman entwined, completely supported by the man—appears frequently in erotic Hindu art. An almost identical position features in the *Kama Sutra*'s repertoire, this time designed to encourage passion and creativity. Not for the faint-hearted, this can be made easier if she leans against a wall and pushes her back into it for leverage. A favorite show-off position, it's primal and perfect for a quickie (see pages 74–75).

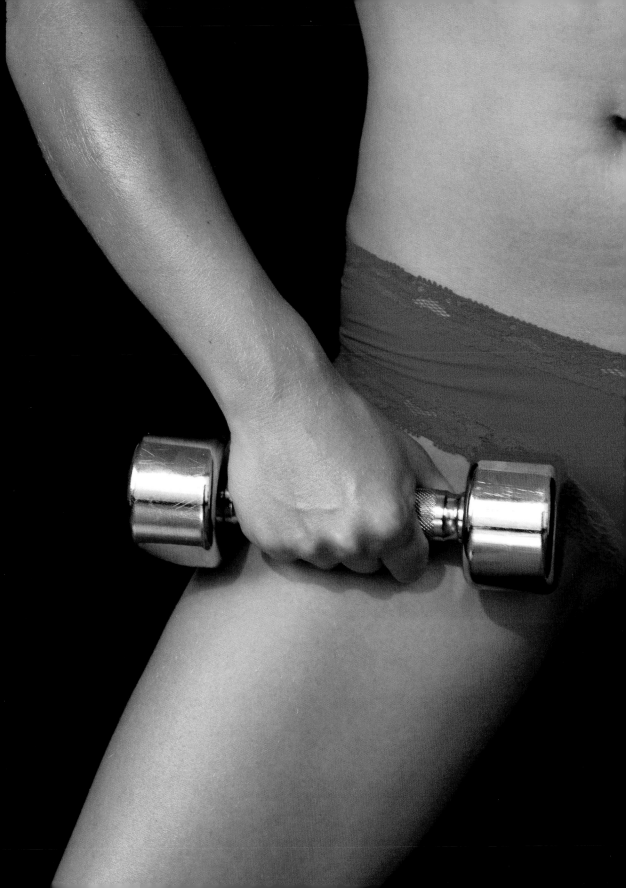

Fit for sex
Healthy body = healthy sex life

So you're looking around the bar, checking out the talent and ready to find someone to try out all those tempting Tantra techniques on, when your eyes settle on the guy in the corner. He's downing his seventh beer, polishing off his third bag of chips, and about to light his 25th cigarette of the day. Sexy beast! Not. But forget the beer gut, pimply skin, bad breath, and stained teeth, they're just the external reasons why this guy isn't a nominee for superhot sex. His poor diet and unhealthy lifestyle make him lethargic—and you need energy for good sex. He's also more likely to have erection problems because smoking has been linked to impotence and a low libido, given that he's starved of desire-enhancing nutrients. Tantric, Tao, Kama Sutra—all three schools of thought work on a holistic approach to sex. To get sex right, everything needs to work together as a well-coordinated whole. That means taking care of yourself spiritually, emotionally, and physically. Here's how...

EAT YOUR WAY TO BETTER SEX

There's always been a link between food and sex, but quite apart from its obvious hedonistic pleasures (eaten, smeared, or inserted!), it's the nutrients that are essential for good sex. The better your diet, the more energy you have to do naughty things. The better your body image, the more inclined you'll be to show your body off. Skipping meals makes us irritable; overeating makes us feel fat, sluggish, and deeply unsexy. The trick to maintaining your sex drive, feeling and looking good, and keeping your libido hovering deliciously high, is to eat little and often, and include lots of "sexy" foods in your diet. While all healthy food is good for you, some nutrients are linked to sexual health more than others. Ian Marber (The Food Doctor and wonderful friend) suggests you add the following to your shopping cart to keep everything in a tip-top sexual state:

- **Zinc:** The most important mineral for sexual behavior and fertility, zinc helps create enzymes that govern taste and smell—both crucial for sexual arousal. Boost your levels with shellfish, eggs, cheese, lamb, poultry, lentils, brown rice.
- **Magnesium:** This keeps your sex hormones nicely balanced, aids sexual stamina, and is vital for sexual sensitivity, arousal, ejaculation, and orgasm. Boost your levels: eat green leafy vegetables, nuts, cheese, bananas, cereal.
- **Calcium:** We need it for nerve transmission and muscle contraction associated with male erection and female orgasm. Boost your levels: eat dairy products, green leafy vegetables, beans, prunes, nuts, dried fruit.
- **Arginine:** This amino acid derived from protein foods is necessary for all growth and sexual development. Boost your levels: eat all animal foods, dairy, popcorn (yes, really).

Our sex life mirrors the rest of our life. It's a reflection of our health, lifestyle, emotions, and relationships. The better they are, the better sex we're having.

- **Vitamin C:** Not just for guarding against the common cold, it also boosts your sex drive and strengthens the sex organs. Boost your levels: eat berries, citrus fruits, mangoes, potatoes, broccoli.

ADD A SEX SUPPLEMENT:

- **Natural Viagra:** The amino acid L-arginine is generally regarded as the natural equivalent of Viagra and is a much safer alternative if you have high blood pressure. It works by increasing the level of a chemical called nitric oxide in the body. This acts as a nerve transmitter, increasing blood flow to the penis. It's found in chicken, eggs, beef, and dairy products, or you can take concentrated quantities in a supplement. Yohimbe is another alternative. It was prescribed for erectile dysfunction before Viagra became available.
- **Good for guys:** Siberian ginseng (increases sperm count), yerba mate (for short-term energy), sarsaparilla (for prostate health), saw palmetto (for erection problems).
- **Good for girls:** Evening primrose oil (for PMS and a high sex drive), bee pollen, and royal jelly (both also boost sex drive); catuaba (reduces stress), chaste berry (regulates hormones).

The body's production of feel-good endorphins can increase up to 200 percent from the beginning to the end of a good

SEXERCISE

Any woman who's ever had a child knows all about "Kegel" or "PC" exercises. Seems like you've just finished pushing the baby out when the doctor starts telling you to pull everything in again. (Like, *owwwww!*) As much as you'd be justified in telling the doc to get lost when you're still at the stage

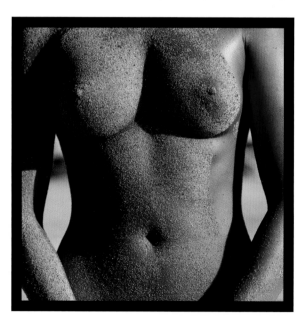

when you swear you'll never have sex again, regularly contracting your vaginal muscles is such an effective exercise, you'd be well advised to smile sweetly and listen up instead. Pelvic floor exercises don't just produce a tight vagina (which, by the way, isn't just for him, it increases your sensitivity as well), they also boost sexual desire, intensify orgasm, and can help you become multi-orgasmic. Sound good? Let's start squeezing!

First, find your PC muscle by stopping the flow of your urine (try not to pull in your bottom or tummy at the same time). Once you've isolated it, squeeze and contract, holding it for a few seconds, then release.

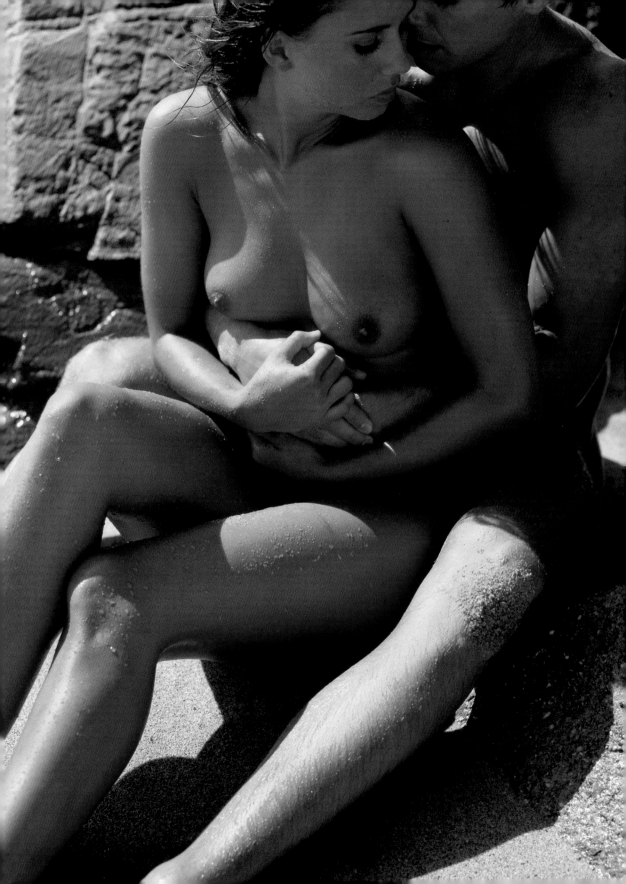

Start with repetitions of 25 and do two sets a day. It's then a case of working up to around 50 repetitions, several times a day, but holding the squeeze for longer. That's your basic exercise, but if you really want to make a difference fast, take a tip from *The Multi-Orgasmic Woman* (by Mantak Chia and Dr. Rachel Carlton Abrams) by doing the following routine—it gets excellent results, trust me!

- Lie down or sit on the edge of the bed or chair and insert two fingers inside your vagina, up to your second knuckle.
- Squeeze your PC muscle around your fingers. Hopefully, you'll feel your vagina contract around your fingers. (If you don't, do a week or two of basic Kegel exercises to get the muscles in shape.)
- Spread your fingers apart to make a "peace" sign, but keep them relaxed. Now contract your muscles and try to bring your fingers together, using just the muscle.
- Try contracting and holding for 10 seconds, then relax for 10. Aim to do 10 repetitions, twice a day.

Be realistic: age affects erections. You're not going to be **as hard** or have **as many at age 40** as you did when **you were 18.**

DO PENIS PUSH-UPS

She's not the only one who'll benefit from doing PC exercises. The pubococcygeus muscle in men is a muscular sling that stretches from the pubic bone in the front to the tailbone in the back. Again, find it by stopping your urine in midstream. Chances are you'll probably feel it in the perineum (the area between your testicles and anus). This muscle is also responsible for the contractions you feel in your pelvis and anus during orgasm. Taoists (and others) believe that if you strengthen this muscle enough, you can have multiple orgasms—yes, just like her! Orgasm and ejaculation are two separate processes—orgasm is simply the feeling in the brain. By strengthening your PC muscle, it's possible to control ejaculation and separate the two so you can feel an orgasm in your brain, without ejaculating. For the rest of you, who'd simply like to intensify your orgasms, strengthen your erections, (and be able to show off to your girlfriend by putting a towel on your erect penis and moving it up and down), this exercise will do nicely.

- Isolate the muscle by stopping your urine in midflow.
- Mentally focus, then breathe out, contracting your PC muscle.
- Now breathe in while releasing the muscle.
- Start with 10 repetitions and work up to around 40. You can't overdo this, so aim for at least two or three sets a day. (Yes—a day! And you can't use the "I'm too busy" excuse for this one. The joy of Kegels is that you can do them anywhere without anyone knowing.)

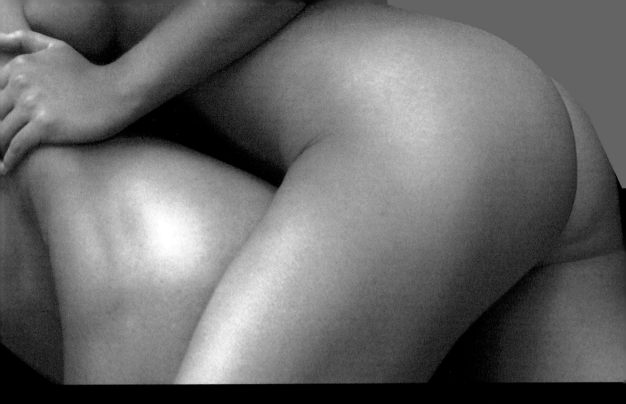

FOR A HAPPY, HEALTHY VAGINA

- Change your tampon frequently.
- To always smell sweet, avoid garlic, tight clothing, synthetic panties, pantyhose.
- Wipe front to back after using the toilet.
- Rinse thoroughly after washing.
- Ideally, wash with a soap-free liquid (available in most drugstores).
- Pee before and after sex to flush out bacteria.
- Don't even think about using vaginal deodorant.
- Have sex a lot to keep your muscles toned and your vaginal walls flexible.
- Masturbate regularly using a variety of techniques (fingers, vibrator) so you don't become dependent on one type of stimulation.
- Use a good-quality lubricant to protect the delicate walls of the vagina from tiny cuts and tears.
- Exercise—it improves the blood flow essential for sexual arousal.
- Stop smoking. It's linked to cervical cancer

FOR A HAPPY, HEALTHY ERECTION

- Be realistic. Age affects erections. You're not going to be as hard or have as many erections at 40 as you will at 18. Don't stress about it.
- Lead a healthy life, and exercise. The better your general health, the less likely you are to need medication—a common cause of erection problems.
- Avoid stress—a calm penis is a happy one. Overworked, exhausted penises (not surprisingly) have trouble rising to the occasion.
- Watch your diet. Burgers, pizza, too much beer—it all works to slow down your blood flow. A strong, regular blood flow is what's needed to engorge the tissues that make your penis get hard.
- Don't binge-drink. One drink gives you courage, another loses your inhibitions, the third often loses your erection.
- Don't smoke. As I said, there are definite links between smoking and impotence.

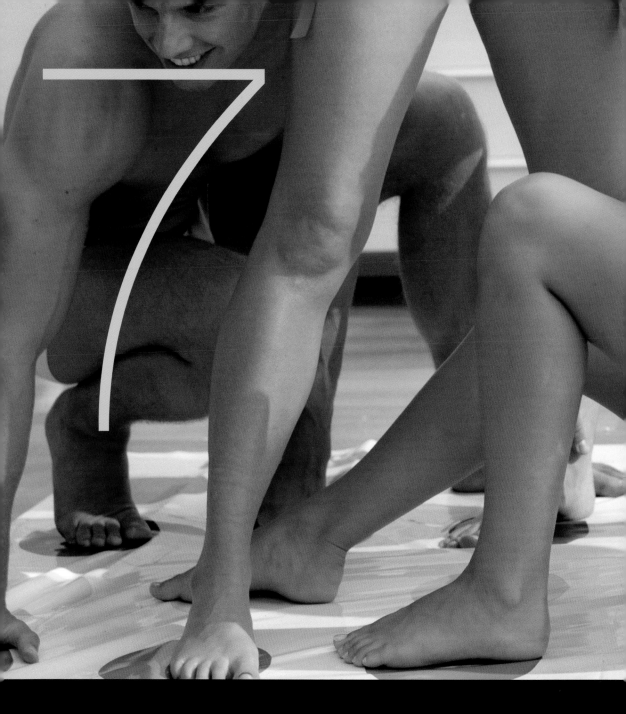

7

saucy games, "treat" techniques and one sensational sex weekend: all you need to make love and make merry! The couple that plays, stays.

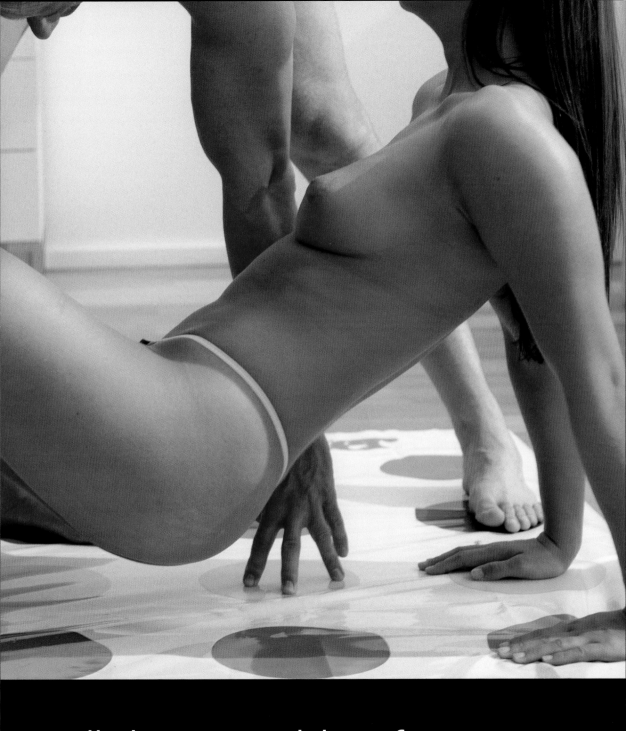

a little something for
the weekend

game for anything

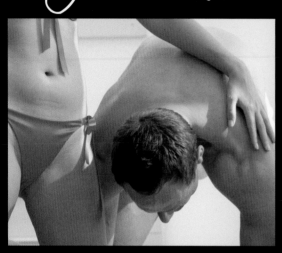

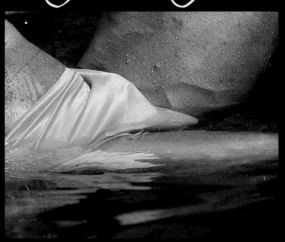

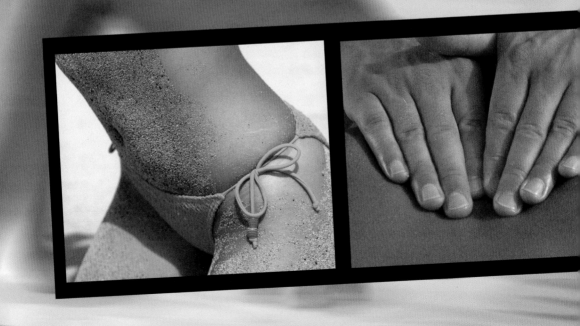

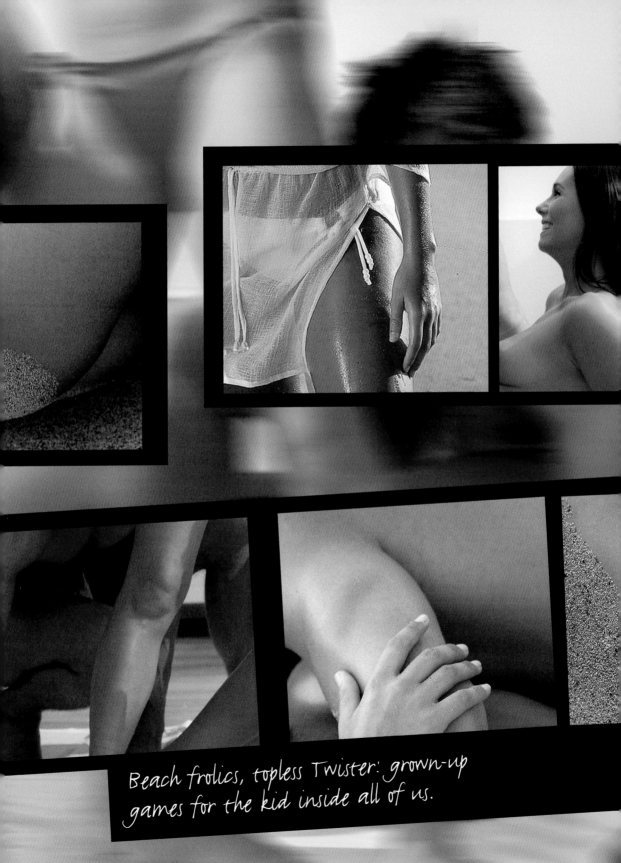

Beach frolics, topless Twister: grown-up
games for the kid inside all of us.

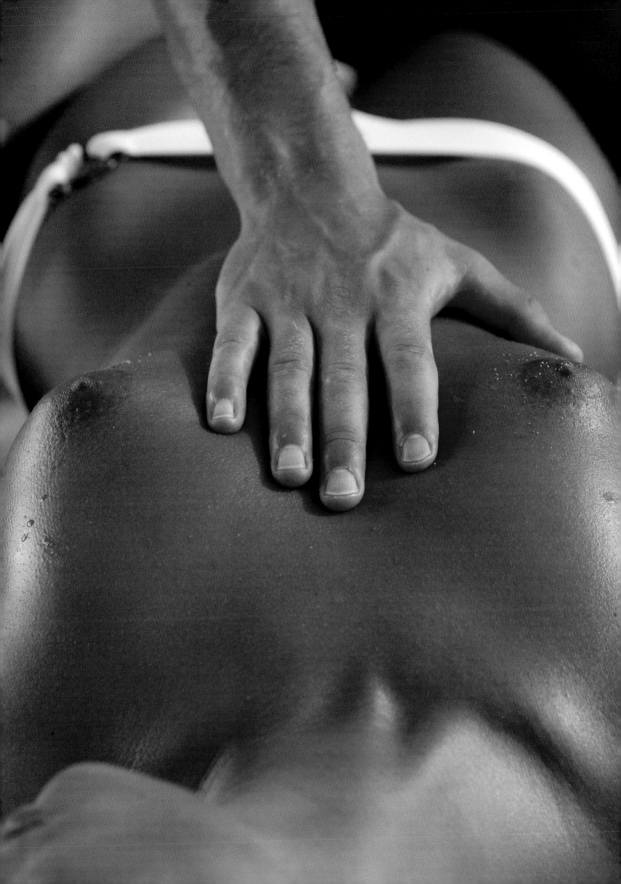

Your sensational sex weekend
Tried, tested, and planned to perfection!

In a recent survey of American marriage counselors, therapists were asked to reveal the one thing they thought most helped save a struggling marriage. Over 80 percent chose regular weekends away. Don't underestimate what two days away from routine, pressure, and normality can do for your relationship and sex life! If you can find a babysitter, escape without the children (squash guilt by

Being **slightly tipsy** at a completely inappropriate time of the day sets the scene for your slide into **complete and utter hedonism!**

reminding yourselves that happy parents = happy kids). If not, choose somewhere the kids can play unsupervised by you. While a fancy hotel is the ideal and most popular choice (the reason why I've used one as a base for this guide), it doesn't need to be expensive. There are amazing deals to be found on the Internet—snap up the bargains by planning ahead and, ideally, aim for one weekend away every two to three months.

One final bit of advice, though, before we get down to the nitty-gritty: remember that the best-laid plans can go astray. Some of my romantic getaways lost their shine when I got food poisoning (too adventurous with local cuisine, too soon), a crippling bout of cystitis (too much sex, too soon), was feeling so sore and swollen that sex was impossible (too much sex, too soon), or was too drunk to have sex (too much, too soon again). (Who me, excessive?) Be prepared for any potential problems by using lubricant, and taking supplies of thrush cream, antibiotics for urinary infections, spare contraceptive supplies, aspirin for hangover headaches, and spare credit cards in case there's a problem drawing money from a particular account.

Right! Now that that's settled, here's a stroke-by-stroke, lick-by-lick, thrust-by-thrust guide of what to do, where, and when. Feel free to adapt the plan to suit your mood and destination, add your own signature sex moves, and I promise this is one weekend you're not going to forget in a hurry!

Saucy underwear is compulsory to pack. So are your favorite sex toys, a scarf for tie-up, a blindfold, massage oil...

DAY ONE: ON THE WAY THERE

On a plane: Drink! I don't care if it's 6 am, your corn flakes are sitting uncomfortably, and your eyes are held open with last night's toothpicks. Pry them wide enough to read the drinks menu and order champagne. Drink it. Lots of it. Being slightly tipsy at a completely inappropriate time of the day sets the scene for your slide into complete and utter depravity and hedonism. (This is a good thing.) If you're a confirmed teetotaller, you're allowed sparkling water, but you *have* to order chocolate to maintain the wickedness level. Skip the mile-high club (overrated—and uncomfortable) and instead place a blanket over your laps and discreetly fool around while one reads and the other looks innocently out of the window.

Turn the TV to the porn channel—it's come a long way since Debbie did Dallas. You might well find there's a **smattering of smart, sexy, female-produced erotica** nestled among the traditionally tacky stuff.

In a car: Getting a blow-job while driving fast along a highway in a convertible (car—red; girl—blonde) is up there on most men's "What I *Really* Want For Christmas" list. But there's a reason why this fantasy tends to be fulfilled by cheerleaders and college girls: when you're 18, you tend not to think things like "If he's having an orgasm, he's not exactly paying attention to driving" or "This could be fun but could also kill us." A less dangerous, but no less appealing version of this, is to casually reach across, unzip and expose him, then dispense a leisurely, lazy hand-job that keeps him standing to attention but not losing it.

On arrival: Explore the hotel, "ooh" and "aah" at all the nice things—then choose one place in the room that particularly strikes you. This is the location for some teasing. She gets two minute-long bouts of oral sex (broken by kissing her breasts). He gets two minute-long bouts of fellatio (broken by kissing his neck). Don't remove all your clothes, just pull your panties aside and his pants to his knees. You're not allowed full sex yet (and no, I won't be bribed!).

During the day: After lunch and perhaps some shopping, go for a walk in the countryside/around the resort and have sex somewhere you might get caught. There's an exhibitionist trapped inside all of us. When we were young, we quickly learned that anything our parents banned was a hell of a lot of fun. As an adult, the law bars us from doing sexy things outside or in public places, so we automatically assume that'll be great as well. And it is! To openly defy the rules feels fabulous! It might take you a few swift ones to get up the nerve, and you might feel slightly appalled that you took the risk in the cold light of the next day. But at that very second, it's worth every heart-stopping

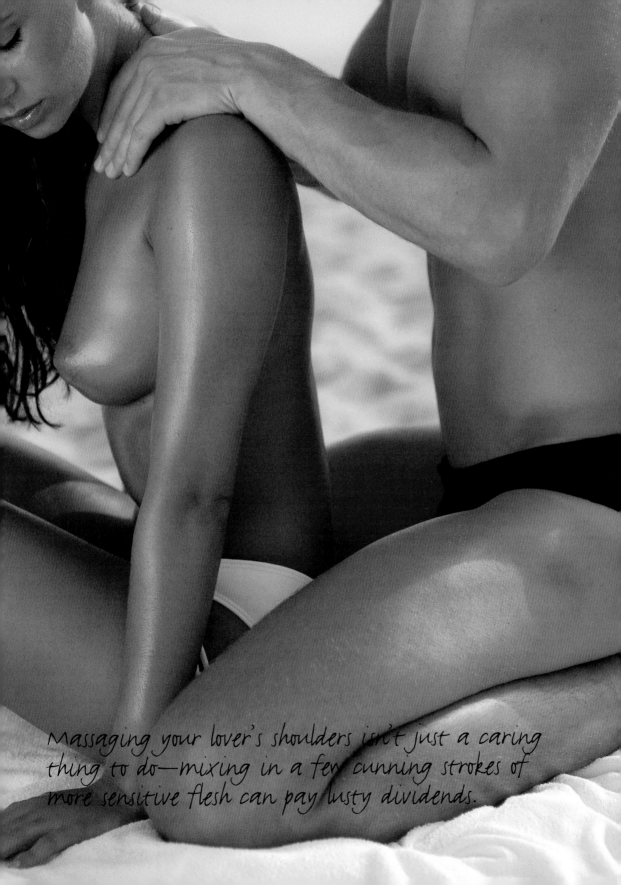

Massaging your lover's shoulders isn't just a caring thing to do—mixing in a few cunning strokes of more sensitive flesh can pay lusty dividends.

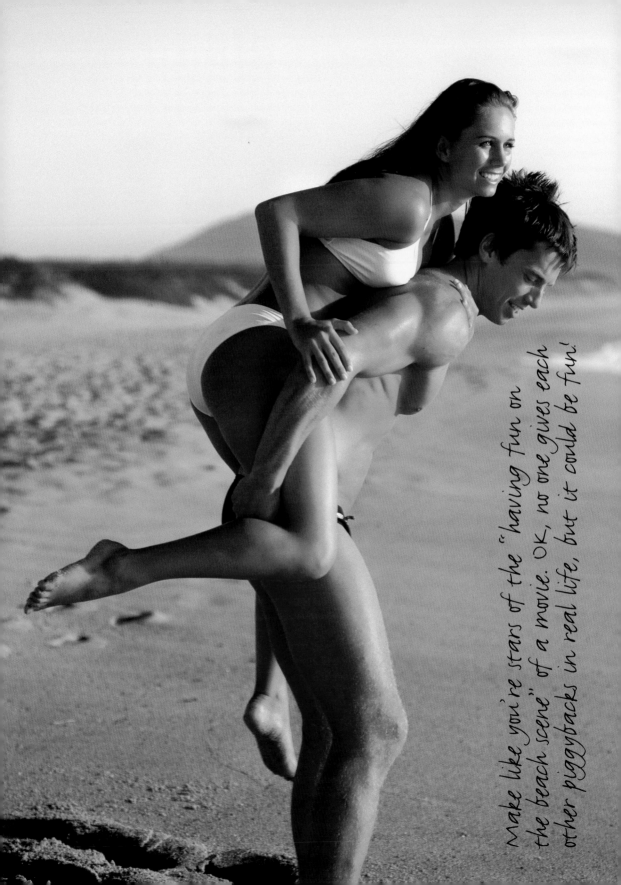

Make like you're stars of the "having fun on the beach scene" of a movie. OK, no one gives each other piggybacks in real life, but it could be fun!

moment. If you're too chicken (or in a country where the penalty for even kissing outdoors is to be beheaded), capture the sense of being discovered by doing it on the balcony where passers-by can only see your seemingly innocent top half.

After dinner: Turn the TV to the porn channel—it's come a long way since Debbie did Dallas. While traditional porn still features heavily, there's usually a good smattering of new stuff, some made by women for women. In other words, there are X-rated movies out there that are smart, fun, and clever. Keep in mind that most porn is highly doctored, porn stars are chosen for extreme appendages, and nearly all the sex is highly unrealistic (women orgasm in seconds at the sight of a man's thigh), and you might find it's arousing (not to mention a good laugh). Make it even more fun by enforcing a rule as you're watching: you can touch your partner but they can't touch you. Then swap roles.

DAY TWO

Wake your partner by kissing them, then put your hands over their eyes, effectively robbing them of their sense of sight. Make it more permanent by using a blindfold (such as a scarf or the "sleep mask" you got on the plane). Being blindfolded and made love to is a top turn-on for many because it sends anticipation skyward. You might think you know your lover's moves inside out, but if you're not sure what you're getting, where and how, predictable turns startlingly sexy.

After your afternoon nap: Play strip dice. List the numbers one to six and make each number correspond to clothing (1. jeans 2. bra. 3. socks etc.). Then take turns throwing the dice. Depending on which number comes up, the thrower has to take off the corresponding item of clothing. But you can't just remove it—it has to be done striptease-style, flamboyantly and dramatically!

Drinks before dinner: Pre-dinner cocktails are enjoyed in your room, looking at the view (each other) and having a kissathon. If you don't really like how your lover kisses, this is a good way to get them to change, without having to ask outright. Instead, challenge them to a kissing competition where you both have to see how many different techniques you can come up with. Be particularly enthusiastic of the technique you most like and even the dimmest lover usually gets the hint.

Back in bed: Make like you're a mannequin. One of you becomes a store dummy, unable to move. The other has a field day—kissing, fondling, touching, and penetrating. You can play this game two ways: simply as a teasing game or as a form of erotic feedback. In the second version of the game, the "mannequin" still can't move but can speak, calling out a number from one to ten to rate how good the sensation feels.

Become narcissists:
- Most hotels discreetly position full-length mirrors so you can watch yourselves in bed. Position yourselves so the person receiving pleasure can see exactly what's going on.
- If your room has a large bathtub, it's rude not to have sex in there! Go easy on the bubbles so you have a good view of gloriously naked flesh. Pick favorite parts of your partner's body—look but don't touch as you wax lyrical.

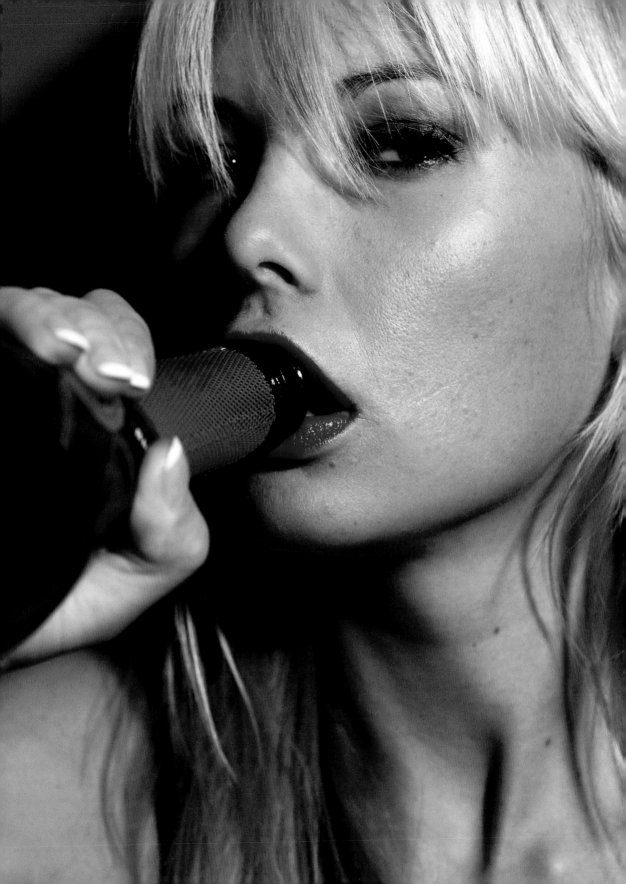

Great sex games
Because grown-ups need fun too!

Some people love games, others loathe them. But even if you are the type who develops sudden diarrhea at the mere mention of the word "charades," you might just find something to tickle your fancy here. As I always say (over and over and over, till you're sick of hearing it): the couple that plays together, stays together. The reason I keep repeating myself is this: *it's true*!! Stop playing and you'll fall out of love. Keep having fun and you'll stay together. Simple as that. Now, do as you're told. I order you to have fun!

> Stop playing and you'll fall out of love. Keep having fun and you'll stay together. Simple as that. **Having fun isn't a luxury, it's essential.**

TO HAVE A BIT OF A LAUGH

• **Make obscene phone calls:** One of you goes outside or into another room, then dials the other, pretending they have no idea who they've just called—but have every intention of being shockingly rude. Ask questions like: "What are you wearing?" Give instructions like: "Pull your panties to one side for me," "Reach down and grab that big, sexy erection you've got." At first, the person you've called is shocked and outraged, but then they seem oddly turned on by it all...

• **Be flashers:** Turn the lights off, then take turns lighting one area of your own body with a flashlight. Each lit body part must be touched, stroked, and/or licked for two minutes, then the light gets passed on to the next person. (Note to boys: It gets very, very boring if the only thing ever under the spotlight is long and cylindrical.)

• **Play "dress-up":** Vinyl nurses' outfits, baby doll lingerie, all-in-one catsuits—they're straight out of the 80s and tons of fun. You pay through the nose for them in a sex shop and they're not terribly well made, but if you have a little cash and you like them, why not? If the thought of you dressed up as Nurse Betty/Spiderman makes you want

If you're noisy types, record yourselves having sex. Play it back when you're somewhere you can't fool around. It's one hell of a turn-on....

to scream with hilarity rather than lust, put together a less obvious home-spun creation. For her, a little kimono with nothing underneath, or long black satin gloves worn with a push-up bra, or high heels and no panties. For him, a bare chest with a pair of great jeans, top button undone, or a fetching pair of testicle-hugging Calvins.

TO LEARN MORE ABOUT EACH OTHER'S HOT SPOTS

- **Fantasy dice:** Write down and number the beginning of six fantasies (something like "Suddenly I felt my girlfriend's mother put her hand on my knee under the table. Even worse, she was really attractive" or "And there I was—in the middle of an orgy"), then take turns throwing the dice. When the person lands on a number, they have to complete the corresponding fantasy out loud. It's a sneaky, not-too-embarrassing way to find out your partner's secret turn-ons because we rarely make up a fantasy that doesn't appeal to us.

Make up your own redeemable sex coupons and leave promised treats for your partner to discover. **Their reward for being very, very good is your being very, very bad.**

- **Be a sex therapist:** One of you goes somewhere private to take a call from a "patient" you're trying to help. The patient rings and pretends to ask for advice on how to please their partner. The therapist goes into lots of detail describing what would be a good way to do this. (All, of course, their personal idea of heaven!) If you like this one, get the therapist to make an appointment for the patient, so the therapist can give "hands-on" demonstrations of each technique.

- **Look, no hands!** There's a tendency for people to do most what they think they're best at, and if you're too dependent on your hands to turn each other on, cut them off! Or perhaps not. A less drastic option is to tie your partner's hands together, then ask them to seduce you. They've got no option but to up the oral quotient by using their lips, teeth, and tongue—or inventively explore interesting options using parts of themselves they wouldn't usually dream of incorporating into love play. If you really want to make things interesting, *both* of you tie your hands behind your backs.

- **Play guinea pig:** Grab all the sex toys you own (order some new ones if there's a lone vibrator lying forlornly in the drawer—there are loads of couple-friendly products out there for you to try), then place them on a table in the bedroom, lined up in a formal fashion. Tell your partner they're needed as a "test dummy" for a project you're working on that night. Strip them naked and try out each and every toy on them. They have to rate them in order of pleasure.

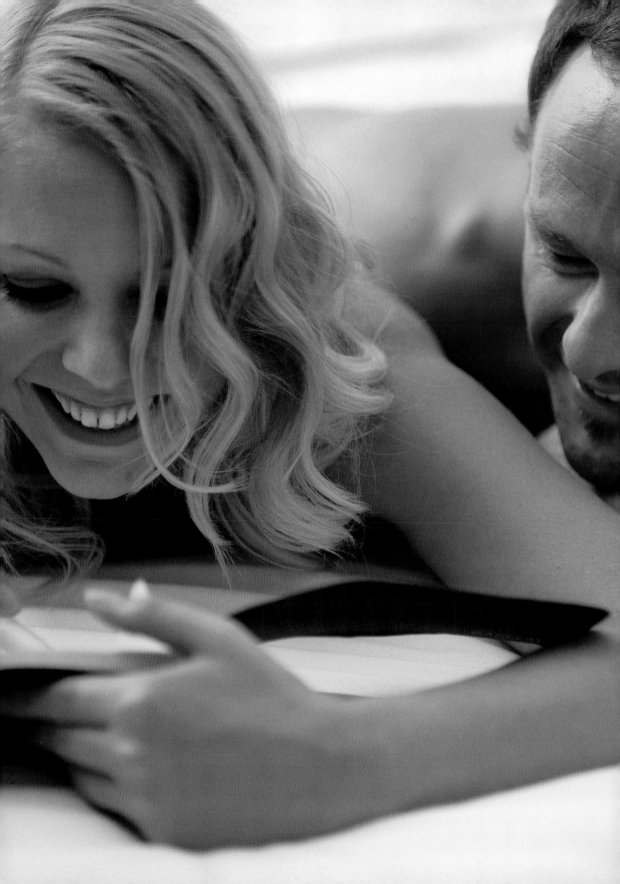

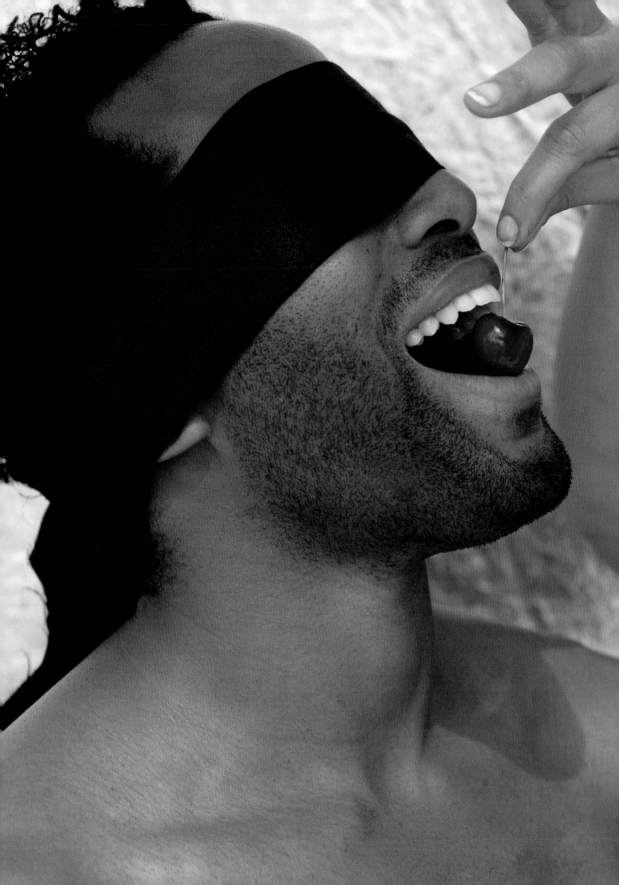

BANISH BORING, ROUTINE SEX

Play cards: There are loads of saucy playing cards around, with everything from cutesy to plain pornographic images pasted on the back. Use these to play any traditional card game. There are others, however, that don't just offer a visual treat, they also provide a novel way of improving your sex life in a nonthreatening format. *supersexdeck* is my card game (blush), which includes cards that have an intercourse position on the front with info on how to get the best out of it on the back. Pick a card, any card, and that nasty him-rolling-on-top-after-a-six-pack habit could be a thing of the past. There are also cards with sexy pics and tips—all designed to help long-term lovers be more sexually adventurous and new lovers find each other's sexual triggers. If you're shy, they're a godsend. Too embarrassed to tell your partner your needs and desires? Let the cards speak for you! (*supersexdeck* is available from www.traceycoxshop.com).

Play with food: Smear it, insert it, drip it on and lick it off—food is such a versatile sex toy, the possibilities are endless. But don't just think whipped cream, honey, and ice cream. Try warmed chocolate sauce, raspberry syrup—hell, bread-and-butter pudding if that's what does it for you! If you're on a diet (What, even in bed? Really?) go for avocados, mangoes, berries, and bananas. Most foods (bar hot, spicy ones) are safe to smear on the outside of the genitals, but you do need to be a bit careful inserting things. Sugary food can set off yeast infections; oily foods leave a film that has a nasty habit of "eating" condoms because oil breaks down latex. (Why you would want to insert that Italian antipasto platter is beyond me, but just thought I'd warn you.) Never, ever squirt or spray anything into the anus or vagina (not even whipped cream) because it's incredibly dangerous. While it's OK to turn your partner off occasionally when trying new things, turning them off *permanently* isn't the name of the game. Food isn't just for smearing, by the way—some people actually eat it! Jumping into bed together, ready to devour a tray full of decadent goodies, is unbeatably hedonistic. Choose bite-size finger foods that look, taste, and feel sexy: smoked salmon, strawberries, grapes, chocolate, olives, oysters on ice, asparagus.

Put pen to paper: If J.K. Rowling can do it, so can you. OK, perhaps your imagination and storytelling skills aren't quite up to her standard, but give it a shot nevertheless. Make up an erotic story based on you and your partner, fill it with as much detail as possible, then slip it in your partner's pocket/briefcase/handbag or leave it under their pillow at bedtime.

Surprise, surprise
- Wait until your partner is in bed, then get in yourself—from the bottom end. Crawl under the covers, taking pit-stops at places of interest.
- Remember when you couldn't wait to be in private so you could rip each other's clothes off? The minute you walk inside, grab them and flatten them against the wall, *without* turning the lights on first.

The 10 all-time-best oral sex techniques
Master these and they'll love you forever

HIS TOP FIVE

1. Lollipop: This one is often used in porn movies because it lets him see exactly what's going on. To fuel this fantasy, drop to your knees. (Depending on your heights, he might need to stand on something—you need good access to his testicles.) Lift his penis to expose his testicles, then find the line that runs between them (it's a tiny ridge that's often a darker color). Find where this starts on the underside of his testicles, and that's where your lollipop lick starts—continuing, very slowly, to the tip of his penis. Repeat the full-length licks (at least 10), then move into the "classic."

2. The classic: Use one hand to hold the base of the penis and let saliva pool in your mouth (your tongue needs to keep him nice and slippery). Make a loose fist with your other hand and slide it up and down his penis, closing it when you reach the head. Get the hand motion right first, then add your mouth, letting your hand act as an extension of it. Create a snug vacuum (but don't suck), then slide up and down, your hand following your mouth. If you're not the most coordinated person, hold your hand still at the base of the penis and simply move your mouth up and down.

3. The twist and swirl: Add oomph to the "classic" or any oral technique by adding the "twist and swirl." The combination of firm fingers and a soft tongue feels great and it's easy to master. As you're using your hand to masturbate him, twist it slightly once it reaches the head and at the same time, swirl the flat of your tongue around the rim of the head. A simple but oh-so-effective move! Also try frenulum flicks: flicking it using a tensed tongue; or make like a butterfly and "flutter" the frenulum.

4. Ball games: The greatest compliment you can give him is looking like you want to be down there—and one of the best ways to show this is to explore all of him. Take one or both testicles in your mouth, hum lightly, suck gently, and/or swirl your tongue around. (If you don't want to swallow, switching to testicle stimulation while working on him with your hand is a good alternative.)

5. Rimming: Rimming is oral anal stimulation (sometimes called analingus). It involves licking, flicking, or inserting a stiff tongue into the anal passage and thrusting like a pretend penis. It feels great (for both sexes actually) because the area is highly sensitive and loaded with nerve endings. If you're worried about germs, STDs or generally squeamish, put a barrier between it and you—try a piece of plastic wrap, or cut open a condom and lay it across the opening.

A **magic tongue** is one thing, but what you do with your hands can mean **the difference between good oral sex and fan-friggin'-tastic oral sex.**

HER TOP FIVE

1. The classic: Separate the vaginal lips with your fingers, find the clitoris, and lick around the edges, slowly and gently. Then relax your tongue and wiggle it side-to-side and up and down over the clitoris and/or clitoral hood (depending on how sensitive she is). On orgasm, press your flat tongue against the clitoral head, continuing to lick, or simply let her push against you. Don't remove your tongue until she says so—women's orgasms last much longer than yours!

2. The ice-cream cone: Make your tongue flat and wide, like you're licking an ice-cream cone, and start with long, slow, wet licks on the inner lips. Move from this into a swishing motion—imagine you're catching the drips of ice cream. As your tongue swishes randomly, you're now teasing the edges of the clitoris. Next, alternate long, flat, ice-cream licks on or around the clitoris with firm, short, fast licks using a tensed tongue. (If the clitoris shrinks or she pulls away, you're being too rough.) Alternate the techniques, then settle on the one she seems to like the best, continuing it to orgasm.

3. The zigzag: This technique stops you from overstimulating one area and making the clitoris oversensitive. The zigzag involves alternating vertical strokes of the tongue on the bottom of the clitoris, with horizontal strokes across the whole of it. Horizontal strokes are usually more pleasurable, so do about seven of those to one vertical. Once she's highly aroused, add in some diagonal licks. Tilt your head to the side (your ear on her thigh) and using the side of your tongue, start from a low corner point and finish by brushing up against the clitoral head.

4. Hands on: Let your finger follow behind your tongue so she has a contrast of sensation (soft tongue, firm fingers) or put a finger in her mouth. She'll either give it "mini" fellatio or suck it the way she wants you to lick her. Insert a finger inside her vagina and thrust it in and out; reach up and use both hands to play with her breasts. If she likes anal stimulation, try simultaneously putting your thumb inside her anus, a finger into her vagina, and your mouth on her clitoris.

5. Mirror, mirror: Lots of women think their vagina is a weird, purpley, squishy thing. So a guy who looks at it with lust and/or wonder scores big points. In the early and middle stages of oral sex, suddenly pull back, stopping to stare at her genitals, letting your eyes also gaze over the rest of her (gorgeous) body. Only pause for around a minute (and for God's sake, don't do it as she's about to climax!)

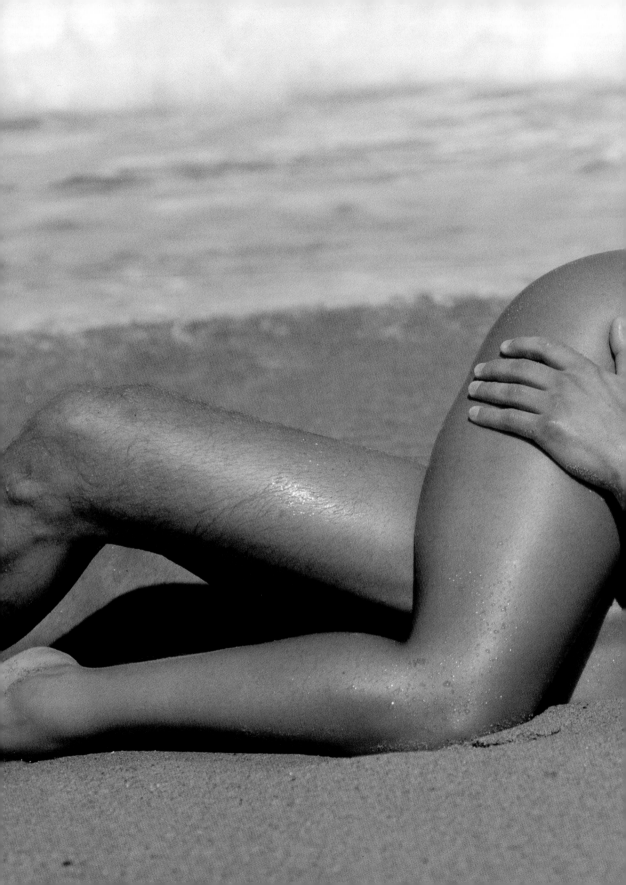

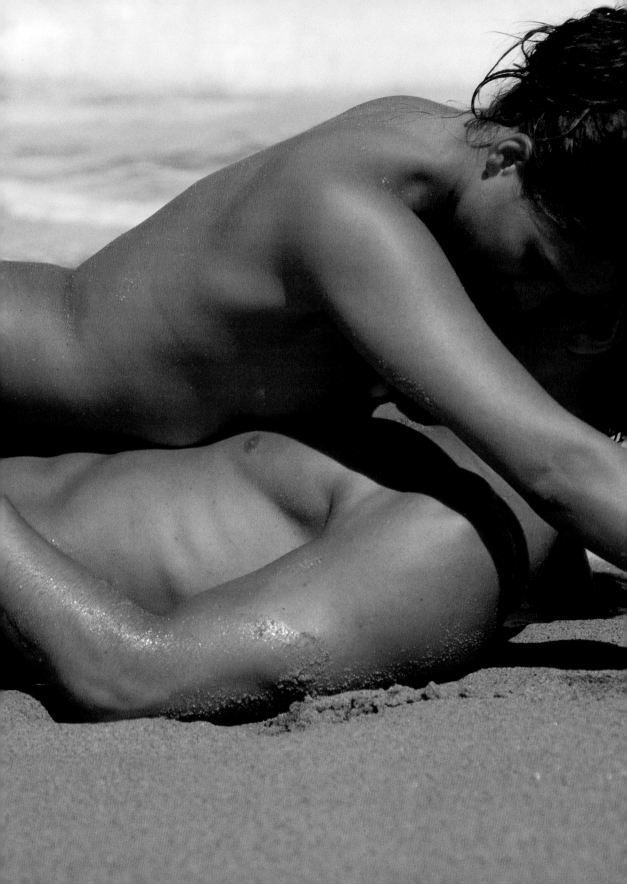

The 10 all-time-best hand-job techniques
Practice makes you the perfect lover

HIS TOP FIVE

Use lubricant for all these techniques—a hand-job without it is like potatoes without the gravy.

1. The classic: This involves wrapping one or two fingers around the shaft of the penis and manipulating the foreskin, so it moves up and down with each stroke. You need to place your fingers exactly where he does at the starting position (ask him to show you how he masturbates). To vary this, make a ring with your index finger and thumb and put it around the base of the penis. As you pull his penis upward, pull the ringed fingers downward to gently pull his testicles away from his body.

2. The favorite: Hold your right hand horizontally in front of you, the back of your hand facing you, thumb pointing downward, elbow cocked. Hold the base of his penis: the back of your hand and four fingers on the side of the penis facing you and your thumb on the side facing him. Slide slowly up the shaft in a firm, continuous movement and when you reach the part where the shaft meets the head, slightly twist your hand. Then, keeping your palm close to the head, twist your wrist to pass your palm over the top of his penis and down the other side. Once you reach the base, slide it back over (in reverse) into the starting position. Repeat with your left hand and keep alternating.

3. Spanish style: Put some lubricant between your breasts, push them together to make a pretend vagina, and let him thrust between them. Not only does it seem wickedly disrespectful (always a good thing in sex, I find!) to be aiming his lethal part straight at your face, he will faithfully follow you around the Pottery Barn every Sunday morning for a month if you let him ejaculate over you.

4. The twist: Imagine you're twisting the cap off a bottle of beer (if you really want to make his day, hand him one before you do this!) Grip the base of the penis with one hand, pulling the foreskin taut, and the head with the other. Now, twist the top hand firmly, return, then twist again, turning it into a continuous motion, slowing down or building up speed depending on his response. Your thumb should be on the frenulum (the stringy bit under the ridge where the head meets the shaft).

5. Finger lock: Clasp your hands and interlock your fingers, overlapping your thumbs, but leaving room for his penis to slip in the middle. Lower your hands over his penis, close your thumbs to take a firm hold, then slide your clasped hands up and down, twisting gently as you do.

Don't finish his hand-job in company unless there's a good airflow. **Semen has a strong, unmistakable smell** and you'll be busted before you can say "God, how embarrassing!"

HER TOP FIVE

As with him, you'll get far better results if you add lubricant for all these techniques.

1. The classic: Place your palm over her pubic hair and bend your middle finger so it's angled ready to touch her clitoris, resting on the inner lips. Position your index and ring fingers so they're resting on the outer lips. Then use your middle finger to gently rub the clitoris up and down or in circles, maintaining a slow, steady rhythm. Squeeze the other two fingers to push the outer lips together and provide extra pressure. A variation is to dip a finger inside her, then slowly slide it along the inner lips of the vagina, moving up toward the clitoris. Let your whole finger roll against the clitoris, then move back down to repeat. Don't touch the clitoris directly the first time.

2. The wall: Put two fingers inside her vagina, then curl them upward so you're pressing against the front wall (as though you're aiming for her stomach). Make sure they're butting up against (or even grab onto) her pubic bone. Massage this top area, using firm pressure, and you're stimulating the "inner clitoris"—the part which is hidden—and the hypersensitive front vaginal wall.

3. Scissors: Put your index and middle finger together, hold them stiff, so they're resting on the inner lips, then move them rapidly from side to side, using a small, gentle movement. Next, "scissor" your fingers, kicking them in alternating directions. Again, keep the movement small or she'll hit the roof with pain, not pleasure.

4. The clock: Imagine there's a clock dial surrounding the clitoris, then work your way around, spending five seconds in each "hour" position, making tiny circles with your fingertips. This ensures you don't overstimulate the clitoris, plus it gets you to concentrate on the edges rather than the center (which most women prefer). Lots of women have a "favorite" side, and you're more likely to discover it this way. To make the feeling more intense, use your other hand to pull up the skin of the mons pubis (fleshy bit). This pulls the clitoris out from under its hood, exposing a larger area.

5. The roll: Use the clitoral hood (the fold of flesh protecting the clitoris) like you would a foreskin, moving it up and down rather than touching the clitoris. Using it as a buffer, roll it between your thumb and index finger to stimulate the clitoris. (You can use the same motion directly on the clitoris.)

Index

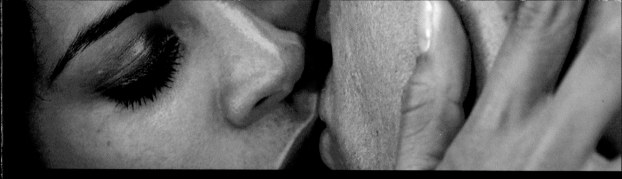

Acknowledgments

This is my ninth book about sex and relationships and I don't know if it's laudable or sad that I still don't feel that I've run out of things to say! One of the reasons I'm never short of material or inspiration is that so many people are willing to share intimate details of their lives with me. For this I am deeply grateful, and while none of you want to be named specifically (can't think why not!), a collective thank-you to all. This is also my ninth list of acknowledgments, and while I have thanked most of the following people previously, my appreciation has grown rather than dwindled over time.

Thank you to my family—Shirley and Terry, Patrick and Maureen, Nigel and Diana, Deborah and Doug, Charlie and Madeleine—who support and encourage me every day of my life.

Thank you to my agent and dear friend, Vicki McIvor, who is as kind as she is clever, and without whom I would be completely and utterly lost.

Thank you to Nigel Wright and Bev Speight of XAB, who work their magic to make all my books look innovative, stylish, and unique.

Thank you to Dawn Bates, who did a brilliant job editing this book and I hope will edit many more.

Enormous thanks to everyone at Dorling Kindersley, worldwide, for being so supportive of all my projects. In the UK office, a huge thank-you to Deborah Wright, Serena Stent, Hermoine Ireland, Liz Statham, Catherine Bell, Adele Hayward, Nicola Rodway, Karla Jennings, Salima Hirani, and extra, extra special thanks to my lovely friend Corinne Roberts. In the US office, Carl Raymond, Therese Burke, Tom Korman, and Rachel Kempster and in Canada, Chris Houston and Loraine Taylor.

Finally, thanks to Pete Collis. You know what for.

DK would like to thank: Alyson Lacewing for proofreading; Valerie Chandler for the index; Stringfellows for their venue; John, Pauline and Olivia Midgley for their Yorkshire location and props; Sh! of Hoxton, London for clothing and props; Lovehoney.co.uk for the sassy, sexy selection of sex toys; IMM Models; Target Models; MOT Models.

Good sex that lasts isn't a gift... it's an achievement.

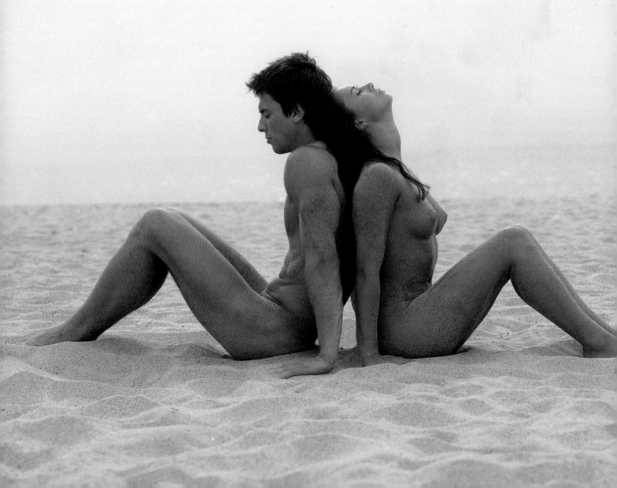